1 MONTH OF
FREE
READING

at

www.ForgottenBooks.com

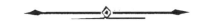

By purchasing this book you are eligible for one month membership to ForgottenBooks.com, giving you unlimited access to our entire collection of over 1,000,000 titles via our web site and mobile apps.

To claim your free month visit:

www.forgottenbooks.com/free278499

ISBN 978-0-266-26258-9
PIBN 10278499

ON THE MECHANISM OF THE PHYSIOLOGICAL ACTION OF THE CATHARTICS

BY

JOHN BRUCE MacCALLUM

Late Assistant Professor of Physiology in the University of California

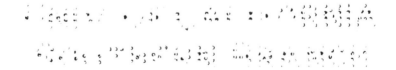

1339

JOHN BRUCE MacCALLUM.

The following pamphlet was completed only a few days prior to the death of the author, which occurred on the sixth of April, nineteen hundred and six. Through his death Physiology was robbed of one of its most brilliant young investigators.

John Bruce MacCallum was born in Dunnville, Canada, on the eighth day of June, eighteen hundred and seventy-six. Through the influence of his father, Dr. G. H. MacCallum, now Superintendent of the State Asylum at London, Ontario, his interest in the natural sciences was early aroused and during his college career at the University of Toronto as much of his time as possible was devoted to these subjects, but chiefly to biology. After his graduation in 1896 he entered the Medical School of Johns Hopkins University. Under the influence of Professor Mall he undertook during his first medical year an investigation on the histogenesis of the cells of the heart-muscle, and it was characteristic of him that he began his work in pathological anatomy also with an original investigation. During the third year of his medical course he again prepared several anatomical papers and at the same time assumed the burden of the proof reading and of preparing the index of Barker's book on Neurology. It was during this year, 1898–1899, that the first symptoms of the disease appeared which was to cut short the life of this talented, indefatigable worker. From this time on he was constantly handicapped in his work by the struggle against illness.

After his graduation in medicine in nineteen hundred he returned to Baltimore as assistant of Professor Mall. In nineteen hundred and one he went to Leipzig to work in the laboratory of His, but his old enemy again interrupted his work, this time attacking him in the form of an affection of the apex of the lungs. He returned home as soon as sufficiently recovered to bear the journey, and upon the advice of Dr. Osler he spent the winter in Jamaica. During this period he translated and edited Szymonowicz's histology into English.

The condition of his health made it impossible for him to live in the East and in the autumn of nineteen hundred and two he went to Denver, "where he rented an office and tried to practice. He abhorred the life, though, and held in contempt the charlatans with whom he came in contact. There were patients and he made enough money to pay his expenses in the few weeks he was there, but the repugnance to that kind of life was too great, and he abandoned his practice. They had made him teacher of anatomy in their medical school, in charge of the department, I believe. The students were difficult to manage—their ideals being far different from his.[1]" The bright spot in his life in Denver was his association with Dr. Sewall, the former physiologist.

Having accepted a call to the University of California, I offered Dr. MacCallum a position as assistant in physiology, and we began our work here together. During the first and second years his health was tolerably good, but in nineteen hundred and five he undertook a problem on immunity which was beyond his physical strength and he began to fail rapidly. He went East to be treated by Professor Osler, returning to Berkeley in the fall of the same year, in a much weakened condition, but if he realized how critical was his condition he betrayed it to no one. He was cheerful and apparently hopeful. As he was not able to exert himself in

---

[1] Quoted from a letter from his brother, Professor W. G. MacCallum, of Johns Hopkins University, to whom I am under obligation for the data given in this sketch.

experimental work, I suggested that he put the results of his experiments done at Berkeley into book form.

The present volume is the result of this work, the last done before death claimed him. It has been published without alteration. The preface was probably written two days before his death, which came suddenly—as he had always wished that it might.

MacCallum belonged to that type of scientists whom we may designate as discoverers. His results were obtained quickly, were made secure beyond doubt, and were put into such shape that they could easily be demonstrated by him. But as is also common in the case of discoverers, his publications were comparatively brief. This may make it at times difficult for inexperienced or uncritical workers to repeat his experiments. I may state, however, that they belong to the regular class exercises of the medical students in our laboratory. Those who have once learned how to perform them can always count upon their succeeding.

In his work as well as in his life he was a calm thinker, the reverse of a hustler. He conceived his experiments in the spirit of an artist and the realization of his ideas was the poetry his work put into his life. He did not work for outside success, nor did he pose as a benefactor of mankind.

Those who have known him well feel that the death of John Bruce MacCallum has left a gap which will never again be filled.

JACQUES LOEB.

BERKELEY, November 7, 1906.

PUBLICATIONS BY JOHN BRUCE MacCALLUM.

1. Fresh-water Cladocera.
    University of Toronto Quarterly, May, 1895.

2. On the Histology and Histogenesis of the Heart Muscle Cell.
    Anatomischer Anzeiger, Bd. XIII, 1897.

3. On the Pathology of Fragmentatio Myocardii and Myocarditis Fibrosa.
    Johns Hopkins Hospital Bulletin, No. 89, 1898.

4. On the Histogenesis of the Striated Muscle Fibre and the Growth of the Human Sartorius Muscle.
    Johns Hopkins Hospital Bulletin, Nos. 90-91, 1898.

5. A Contribution to the Knowledge of the Pathology of Fragmentation and Segmentation and Fibrosis of the Myocardium.
    Journal of Experimental Medicine, Vol. IV, 1899.

6. Development of the Pig's Intestine.
    Johns Hopkins Hospital Bulletin, Vol. XII, 1901.

7. Notes on the Wolffian Body of Higher Mammals.
    American Journal of Anatomy, Vol. I, 1902.

8. On the Muscular Architecture and Growth of the Ventricle of the Heart.
    Johns Hopkins Hospital Reports, Vol. IX, 1900.
    (Memorial volume to Dr. W. H. Welch by his pupils.)

9. Text-book of Histology and Microscopic Anatomy. By L. Szymonowicz. Translated and edited by J. B. MacCallum. Lea Bros., 1902.

10. On the Mechanism of the Action of Saline Purgatives, and the Counteraction of their Effect by Calcium. (A preliminary communication.)
    University of California Publications, Physiology, Vol. I, 1903.

11. On the Action of Saline Purgatives in Rabbits and the Counteraction of their Effect by Calcium. (Second communication.)
    American Journal of Physiology, Vol. X, 1903.
    Also: University of California Publications, Vol. I, 1904.

the Local Application of Solutions of Saline Purgatives to the Peritoneal Surfaces of the Intestine.
American Journal of Physiology, Vol. X, 1904.
Also: University of California Publications, Vol. I, 1904.

the Influence of Calcium and Barium on the Flow of Urine. (A preliminary communication.)
Ibid., 1904.

e Influence of Saline Purgatives on Loops of Intestine Removed from the Body.
Ibid.

e Secretion of Sugar into the Intestine Caused by Intravenous Saline Infusions.
Ibid.

ıe Action of Cascara Sagrada. (A preliminary communication.)
Ibid.

ıe Influence of Calcium and Barium on the Secretory Activity of the Kidney. (Second communication.)
University of California Publications, Physiology, Vol. II, 1904. Also in the Journal of Experimental Zoology, Vol. I, 1904.

ɜber die Wirkung der Abführmittel und die Hemmung ihrer Wirkung durch Calciumsalze.
Pflüger's Archiv, Bd. 104, 1904.

ıe Action on the Intestine of Solutions Containing two Salts.
University of California Publications, Vol. II, 1905.

ıe Action of Purgatives in a Crustacean (*Sida Crystallina*).
Ibid., 1905.

ı the Diuretic Action of Certain Haemolytics, and the Action of Calcium in Suppressing Haemoglobinuria. (A preliminary communication.)
Ibid., 1905.

ıe Diuretic Action of Certain Haemolytics and the Influence of Calcium and Magnesium in Suppressing the Haemolysis. (Second communication.)
Ibid., 1905.

AUTHOR'S PREFACE.

The following pages contain an account of a long series of experiments made to determine the action of saline purgatives. Many of the results have been separately published in various scientific journals, and they are now gathered together with certain new material in an attempt to give as connected and complete an account as possible of the action of this class of drugs.

The experiments were begun at the suggestion of Professor Loeb, to whom I am greatly indebted for the constant interest which he has taken in the work, and whom it is a pleasure to thank for many helpful suggestions.

CONTENTS.

PAGE

Chapter   I.—Normal Movements and Secretion of the Intestine   1

Chapter   II.—The Subcutaneous and Intravenous Injection of Saline Purgatives   9

Chapter   III.—The Local Application of Saline Solutions to the Peritoneal Surfaces of the Intestine 23

Chapter   IV.—The Production of Increased Secretion of Fluid into the Intestine by the Saline Purgatives...... 29

Chapter   V.—The Inhibiting Action of Calcium and Magnesium on the Movements and Secretion of the Intestine 3S

Chapter   VI.—The Action of Saline Solutions on Loops of Intestine Removed from the Body 50

Chapter   VII.—The Action on the Intestine of Solutions Containing Two Salts 57

Chapter VIII.—The Effect on the Intestine of Intravenous Saline Infusions 65

Chapter   IX.—Mode of Action of the Saline Cathartics 74

Chapter   X.—Possible Therapeutic Value of These Experiments 83

Chapter   XI.—The Action of Purgatives of Vegetable Origin...... 86

CHAPTER I.

Normal Movements and Secretion of the Intestine.

A. *Normal Movements of the Intestine.*

The normal movements of the intestine have been described by many observers, and in these descriptions there is a fair amount of uniformity. Ludwig and his pupils, Bayliss and Starling, Magnus and others have studied this subject with much care. In such a complicated organ as the intestine there are many sources of error, and differences of opinion may readily arise if an attempt is made to analyze too closely the functions of the various tissues making up the intestine, to decide for example whether the movements are of nervous origin or muscular, or whether the secretion is dependent primarily on the blood supply or on the nervous system. For our purpose it will be sufficient to regard the intestine as an organ composed of certain muscular layers, certain nervous plexuses and certain glands —and to discuss the action of various influences not on these separate tissues, but on the organ as a whole, holding in mind also the nervous and bloodvascular connections of the organ.

If the abdominal cavity of a dog, cat, or rabbit be opened under the surface of m/6 NaCl solution or Ringer's solution at body temperature, it will be found that the intestines are not entirely at rest. According to local conditions, more or less active movements will be seen. These were described by Ludwig and others as consisting of two kinds of motion, namely, the *pendulum movements,* and *peristaltic movements.*

The pendulum movements are rhythmical, and consist of a regular slight swinging of the loops upon one another. Their frequency has been measured by Bayliss and Starling.[1] According to these observers, each contraction and relaxation lasts 5 to 6 seconds, so that the rhythm consists of 10 to 12 beats per minute. The rhythm is however not always regular, the contents of the loop and other local conditions exerting an influence. The cause of these pendulum movements is not perfectly clear. By many they have been ascribed to a rhythmical shortening of the intestine, *i.e.,* a rhythmical contraction and relaxation of the longitudinal muscle coat. Mall[2] regards them as arising mainly in the circular layer; while Bayliss and Starling state that they are due to simultaneous contractions of the circular and longitudinal coats.

The peristaltic movements consist of more or less strong contractions of the circular coat of the intestine, varying from a slight ring-like contraction which passes rapidly down the gut to a violent constriction of the intestine which obliterates the lumen of the gut and passes very slowly from above downward. The slight contractions may travel, according to Bayliss and Starling, as rapidly as 2–5 cm. per second, while the more violent ones move not more than 1/10 cm. per second. According to Nothnagel, Mall, and others, the formation of these peristaltic waves is always due to a local stimulus, usually the presence of a bolus of food. The intestine contracts immediately above the point of stimulation and the mass of food is forced downward. The wave of contraction follows close behind the bolus, while for some distance above this point similar waves run downward until they reach the mass of food. The gut is usually relaxed below the bolus, and the general statement

[1] Journal of Physiology, Vol. XXIV, 1899, p. 99.
[2] Johns Hopkins Hospital Reports, Vol. I, 1896.

has been made that a stimulation at any point causes a contraction above that point and an inhibition below it. It is generally thought that Auerbach's plexus is concerned in the propagation of the peristaltic wave since the peristalsis takes place also when the intestine is separated from the central nervous system, and does not occur when nicotine or cocaine is given to paralyze the intrinsic nerves of the intestine.

In addition to the pendulum and the peristaltic movements, there is a third quite distinct motion to be observed in the intestine. The normal peristaltic movements are very slow, while this third type, called by Nothnagel "Rollbewegung," consists of a rapid contraction which may pass from one end of the intestine to the other in 1 to 2 minutes. The function of this movement is thought to be the rapid elimination of irritating substances from the intestine. It occurs irregularly and is more common in slight pathological conditions of the gut.

It is generally believed that the normal peristaltic wave passes only from above downward, and never in the reverse direction. This has been shown in many ways. Mall[3] removed a certain length of the small intestine and reversed it so that the end which had originally been nearer the stomach was now in the position formerly occupied by the end nearer the rectum. The food would not pass down this part of the intestine, but accumulated above it. In other words, the peristalsis continued as it was before the loop was removed, the wave passing in the reversed loop from below upward. A further illustration of the same thing is seen in the fact that in an isolated loop an object inserted in the gastric end of the loop will rapidly be passed to the other end, while it is impossible to force the object into the rectal end because of the peristaltic waves which constantly expel it. Grützner[4] observed that the intestinal contents

[3] *Loc. cit.*
[4] Deutsch. Med. Wochenschr., XV, 1899.

sometimes move backward and forward in the intestine, and that an easily recognizable substance, *e.g.*, food introduced into the rectum *in enemata*, was sometimes to be found afterwards in the stomach. It seems further from Cannon's[5] study of the cat's intestine by means of the Röntgen rays that antiperistalsis certainly takes place in the colon of this animal. In the transverse and ascending colon antiperistaltic waves occur at the rate of 5–6 per minute. No antiperistalsis was observed in the small intestine.

Factors which normally cause or influence the intestinal movements. Although there has been some divergence of opinion on the subject, it is now generally held that anaemia of the intestine causes a cessation of all movements. This has been shown by van Braam-Houckgeest,[6] Mall,[7] and others. Clamping of the aorta, opening of the heart, etc., cause all movements to cease. Hyperaemia of the intestine on the other hand causes active movements to arise. Any conditions which cause a venous engorgement of the intestine bring about intestinal movements. Bokai[8] found that CO_2 is a direct stimulant to the intestine, and that the movements may be stopped by the application of oxygen. Krause and Heidenhain first noticed that when an animal's breathing is stopped the peristaltic movements of the intestine greatly increase, but cease when the breathing is recommenced.

The influence of the intestinal contents upon the movements of the gut was discussed as long ago as 1750 by Foelix.[9]. Among the later authors to treat of this subject is Bokai. In addition to indigestible and irritating substances taken in with the food, there are certain substances ordinarily formed in the intestine by decomposition which

---

[5] Amer. Journ. Physiol., Vol. VI, 1902.
[6] Pflüger's Archiv, VI, 1872; VIII, 1874.
[7] Johns Hopkins Hospital Reports, I, 1896.
[8] Arch. f. exp. Path. u. Pharm., Bd. 23-24.
[9] De Motu peristaltic. intest. Treviris, 1750.

cause peristaltic movements. Among these are CO_2, CH_4, and H_2S. All of these gases which are more or less constantly formed help in keeping up the normal movements of the intestine. Certain faecal constituents have also the same effect. Bokai mentions among these a number of organic acids—lactic, succinic, butyric, formic, propionic, acetic, caproic, and caprylic acids. There is no doubt also that the salts taken in with the food exert a considerable influence.

The intestine is to some extent also under the influence of extrinsic nerves. As shown by Pflüger,[10] the splanchnic nerves exert an inhibitory action on the intestine, so that their section causes intestinal movements and their stimulation brings about a cessation of peristalsis. This has been ascribed by some authors to the vasomotor action of the nerves. Concerning the action of the vagus there has been difference of results. Many experimenters have found that stimulation of this nerve causes contractions of the intestine. Others have obtained no results. If, however, the splanchnics be cut and the inhibitory impulses abolished, stimulation of the vagus gives constant results consisting of a slight inhibitory action followed by an increase of the rhythmical contractions of the intestine.

B. *Normal Secretion Into the Intestine.*

It is probable that under normal conditions a fluid is secreted from the entire length of the intestine, but this fluid undoubtedly differs somewhat in the various parts. The duodenum with Brunner's glands, the jejunum and ileum with the glands of Lieberkühn and the large intestine in which there is a preponderance of mucus cells may be assumed to give secretions which are not identical. The methods which have been used to obtain the succus entericus

[10] Über das Hemmungsnervensystem f. d. peristal. Bewegungen d. Darmes, Berlin, 1857.

for analysis are subject to criticism, and much remains to be discovered with regard both to the mechanism of secretion and the nature of the normally secreted fluid. The most fruitful method has been that instituted by Thiry,[11] and later modified by Vella.[12] This consists of the establishment of a permanent fistula from the intestine through the skin from which the intestinal juice may be gathered after complete healing has taken place. This is commonly known as a Thiry-Vella fistula. In general it has been observed that practically no fluid is secreted into the intestine without a stimulus of some sort. Electrical or mechanical stimulation as well as the introduction of food causes a yellowish fluid to pour into the gut. Pregl[13] has studied the secretion by this method in a lamb. Here he finds a continuous secretion which is increased after the taking in of food. It possesses a distinctly alkaline reaction, and contains carbonates, chlorides, and a considerable quantity of proteid. It also contains urea. For a complete analysis the reader is referred to Pregl's article. The intestinal juice of the lamb has no digestive action on proteids. There was formed from starch paste a fermentable sugar. Cane sugar and maltose were inverted, but milk sugar remained unchanged.

The influence of the nervous system on the secretion of intestinal fluid is very clear. It was found by Moreau[14] that section of the nerves to the intestine brought about a large secretion of fluid into the intestine resembling closely that obtained by a Thiry-Vella fistula. Budge[15] had previously noted that extirpation of the ganglia of the coeliac plexus caused an increase of fluid in the intestine. The results of Moreau, who carried out his experiments with isolated loops, have been repeatedly confirmed, and some question has arisen as to the nature of the fluid secreted, some authors

[11] Sitzungsb. d. k. Akad. d. Wissensch. Wien, 1864, Bd. 1.
[12] Untersuchung. z. Naturl. d. Mensch. u. d. Thiere; 1881; Bd. XIII.
[13] Arch. f. d. gesammte Physiologie, Bd. LXI, 1895, S. 359.
[14] Centralbl. d. Medicin. Wissensch., S. 209, 1868.
[15] Verhandl. d. K. K. Leop. Carol. Akad. d. N., Bd. 19, 1860.

regarding it as a transudation, others as a true secretion. It has been compared by some to the rice water stools of Asiatic cholera, and on account of the analogy with the secretion which pours from the salivary gland after section of the chorda tympani it has been called a paralytic secretion. Landois[16] ascribes the secretion to the cutting of vasomotor nerves which causes circulatory changes so marked that a transudation of fluid occurs. In the leg, however, it has been shown that the normal transudation and lymph formation are not increased by section of the nerves. One would also expect to find oedema of the intestinal wall if this were a process of transudation due to vascular changes. Such oedema does not occur.

The nature of the fluid obtained by section of the nerves to the intestine has been studied by many investigators. Moreau described it as a light yellow clear fluid with a strongly alkaline reaction. Its specific gravity is 1.008. It contains carbonates, chlorides, organic materials and a little urea. According to Hanau,[17] the fluid contains no digestive ferments, although in the dog he found that in the first part of the secretion fibrin was digested to some extent and starch converted into sugar. This he ascribed to the presence of pancreatic juice. Mendel[18] has recently worked on this subject and finds also that the pure paralytic secretion has no digestive action on fibrin, but that there is a slight amylolytic action. Cane sugar and maltose are inverted, while milk sugar is not.

The fact that the paralytic secretion resembles very closely the normal secretion both physically and chemically seems to indicate that it is a true secretion and not a transudation.

Bottazzi[19] has recently found that an extract of the small intestine injected into the blood causes not only an increase

---

[16] Lehrbuch der Physiologie, 10th Ed., p. 360.
[17] Zeitsch. f. Biologie, Bd. 22, 1886, p. 195.
[18] Arch. f. d. ges. Physiol., Bd. 63, 1896, p. 425.
[19] Arch. di Fisiologia, 1904, I, 413.

in the fluid secreted into the intestine, but also an increase in the peristaltic movements. This extract is an aqueous one, the nucleoproteids being precipitated by acetic acid. It thus contains the secretin of Bayliss and Starling and is capable of increasing also the pancreatic secretion. The fluid produced in the intestine was later analyzed by Bottazzi and Gabrieli[20] and proved to be quite similar to the normal intestinal secretion. It is of some interest to note that the intestinal secretion and the pancreatic secretion are simultaneously augmented by the intravenous injection of this extract.

---

[20] Arch. internationales de Physiologie, 1905, Vol. III, II, p. 156.

CHAPTER II.

The Subcutaneous and Intravenous Injection Saline Purgatives.

Although it has long been known that many of th
table purgatives act as well when introduced into the
lation as when taken by mouth, it has generally been
that saline purgatives are inactive when injected eith
cutaneously or intravenously. It has even been claim
they have the opposite effect, causing constipation.
Bernard,[21] however, states that sodium sulphate
purgation when introduced into the circulation, al
he gives no experiments to support the assertion.
heim[22] believed that intravenous injection of purgati
produced no purgation. Rabuteau[23] stated that the
tion of a large amount of sodium sulphate into th
caused constipation in a dog, an experiment which
to prove that the strong solution outside the intestin
drew fluid from the lumen by its endosmotic power.
land[24] advanced the view that all medicines act afte
absorbed into the blood, and that saline cathartics a
taken up into the circulation and stimulate the inte
being later excreted by the intestinal glands. Ca
reported an experiment in which he obtained a pu
action by introducing magnesium sulphate into the s

---

[21] Leçons sur les effets des substances toxiques et médicam
Paris 1857

after this organ had been separated from the intestine by a ligature. It was further found by Vulpian[25] that small doses of magnesium sulphate, but not of sodium sulphate, acted as purgatives when injected subcutaneously. Hay[26] gives an excellent resumé of the literature on this subject. Although he considers it already proven that purgatives do not act when injected subcutaneously or intravenously, he has made a number of experiments to confirm this idea. He was unable to obtain any purgative effect in dogs and cats by the introduction into the blood of 10% Na_2SO_4 or 20% $MgSO_4$. With the subcutaneous injection of these salts, however, a purgative action was sometimes produced. This he attributed to the local irritation of the injection. It will be noted that the conditions of these experiments are by no means ideal. Hay injected directly into the blood a solution of Na_2SO_4, which is approximately twice as strong as a solution of this salt isosmotic with the blood would be. Similarly a solution of $MgSO_4$ isosmotic with the blood would be about 4% (m/6 Sol^n $MgSO_4 + 7 H_2O = 4.1$ g. in 100 c.c.). Hence the solution which Hay introduced directly into the circulation was five times as concentrated as an isosmotic solution. Although it is not clear just what abnormal conditions would be brought about by the injection of such concentrated solutions, it is certain that the normal action of the salt could not be expected under these circumstances. This is further shown by the fact that Hay did obtain a purgative action in some cases when he injected the salt solutions subcutaneously. Here the injury caused by the concentrated solution was only local, and the salt itself was absorbed in small quantities and in more dilute solution into the blood.

In a large number of experiments which have yielded quite constant results I have been unable to confirm the

---

[25] Gazette Médicale, 1873.

[26] Journal of Anatomy and Physiology, Vol. XVI, 1882, and XVII, 1883.

nerally held and supported by Hay that subcu
nd intravenous injections of saline purgatives do
 purgative action.   I have quite constantly fou
h proper conditions these salts do produce increa
sis and also an increased secretion of fluid into
e when introduced directly into the circulation
the skin.   In most cases also an actual passage
vas observed.

eral methods were used in testing the action of
d it was found that the results could best be stud
rving the loops of intestine directly.   In rabl
he influence of morphine (5 c.c. 1% solution m
ydrochlorate subcutaneously) the abdominal cav
d open and the loops of intestine carefully protec
ss of heat and moisture while under observation.
ases they were observed under the surface of nor
. chloride solution, a method devised by van Bra
geest and used by him in a long series of experime
NaCl solution the intestines normally remain alm
nd the effect on them of stimulating agents can
 determined. In addition to this method many
nts were made in which animals were kept in se
ges, some acting as control animals, others for
nt.   The amount and character of the faeces w
d during several hours after the administration
gative and compared with the control animals.
as used were made up as fractions of molecular s
Thus to obtain a solution of sodium citrate, for
approximately isosmotic with the rabbit's blood, c
olecular weight of the salt in grams (including wa
tallization) was dissolved in 1,000 c.c. distilled wa
ve an m/6 solution, which was taken to be appr
isotonic with the blood.   The injections were m
 with a hypodermic needle into the marginal vei
bit's ear, or into the jugular vein.   Subcutane

most of these experiments small rabbits weighing from 1,200 to 1,500 grams were used.

In studying the purgative action of these salts, two criteria may be considered, namely, the actual passage of faeces, and secondly merely the increase of peristalsis and secretion not necessarily accompanied by defaecation. The former is of course the object of purgation, and unless a salt produces an actual passage of faeces it cannot strictly be termed a purgative. When this has been established, however, it is of much greater advantage to use the other criterion in studying the action of the solutions on the intestine. Any salt which in small doses produces an increased peristalsis will with a more prolonged action and perhaps larger doses produce actual purgation. Therefore in the first rough test as to the action of the salts I have used the actual passage of faeces as the criterion of the action. In this case no morphine is given the animal and its intestines are not exposed as in the other experiments where the movements are directly watched. In these tests the animals were kept in boxes, the bottom of each of which was covered by a large sheet of paper. During a certain time preceding the injection of any solution the animals were watched and the faeces collected and weighed. Half of the animals were kept as controls, and the rest subjected to injections of various solutions. The average weight of the normal faeces was compared with the weight of the faeces passed during the same time by the animals receiving the injections. The faeces were collected and weighed each hour during the first six hours following the first injection. The chief purgative effect usually took place during the first two hours. Although there was considerable individual variation in the rabbits, there was found to be a constant increase in the amount of faeces following the subcutaneous or intravenous injection of one of the salts. This amount varied from two to six times the average normal weight. Sometimes the increase was much greater and in ιy cases the nature of the faeces was much changed. normal faeces of the rabbit consist of dry hard defily formed masses. Following the purgative, they bee soft and unformed, and may as in the case of NaF and ʔl₂ be semifluid.

The amount of sodium citrate, sulphate, or tartrate ɛssary to produce purgation is about the same in each ʁ: 10 c.c. m/6 solution injected subcutaneously, followed ninutes later by a second injection of 5 c.c. of this solu. and 10 minutes after this by a third similar injection, ally produces well marked passages of faeces. Someɛs the result is obtained with a single injection, but a longed action of the salt seems to be more favorable. ;h sodium fluoride and barium chloride much smaller ɛs are necessary. Sodium fluoride is more poisonous ɑ the citrate or sulphate, but if injected slowly as much 0 c.c. m/6 solution can be safely introduced under the . This produces in a little over an hour well marked gation, usually with the passage of soft or semifluid es. Barium chloride is a well known saline purgative ng veterinary surgeons, who always administer it inenously or subcutaneously. In order to purge a horse hing 1,000 pounds, 0.75 g. BaCl₂ is usually given subneously. Its action is very constant. When given to its I have found that 2 c.c. m/6 solution BaCl₂ injected er the skin always produces a well marked purgative on with the passage of large quantities of semifluid es. When injected intravenously it is better to mix the l₂ with about five times its volume of m/6 NaCl. The etion of 1 c.c. of a mixture of 1 c.c. m/6 BaCl₂ + 5 c.c.

NaCl produces purgation and a passage of semifluid es. This action is much more rapid than with NaF.

These experiments demonstrate the fact that the intraous or subcutaneous injection of saline purgatives do duce purgation and an actual passage of faeces. In er, however, to study the action of the salts more min-

utely another method was resorted to, namely, that of opening the abdomen and directly observing the loops of intestine. In a large number of experiments it is not difficult to
become quite familiar with the movements normally present,
and with the disturbances produced by such external influences as cooling, drying, etc. These influences can by proper
precautions be practically eliminated.

By this method it was possible to study the influence of
the salts on the two great activities of the intestine, namely,
the muscular movements and the glandular activity. Their
action on the secretion is treated of in a later chapter and
can only be mentioned here. The increase of these two
activities by means of a salt is the essential action of a
purgative, and leads, if sufficiently prolonged, to purgation
and to the passage of faeces. This passage of faeces does
not take place so readily when the intestines are exposed
and the animal is under the influence of morphine as it does
in a normal animal. The exposure of the intestine for an
hour or more apparently renders this action difficult, although not uncommonly the actual passage of faeces is observed under these circumstances. This is always the case
with $BaCl_2$.

In a rabbit with its intestines visible it was found that
the injection of 1–2 c.c. m/8 or m/6 sodium citrate solution
into the jugular vein of a rabbit brings about a very marked
increase in the peristaltic movements, which begins from 1
to 2 minutes after the injection. The loops are set in active
movements and become firm and rounded so that they seem
to occupy a greater volume. The movements consist not
only of swinging pendulum movements, but of real peristaltic waves which cause the contents of the intestine to
move along the gut so that they may be watched through the
thin walls. The morphine narcosis of the animal does not
seem to interfere with this action of the salt.

When these salt solutions are administered subcutaneously they do not act at once, as in the case of intra-

venous injections. An interval of 10 to 15 minutes elapses after the subcutaneous injection before any influence on the intestine is noticed. The movements then begin as before, the peristaltic movements and pendulum movements gradually increasing in force. In addition to the greater time required for the action of the salt when administered in this way, it is also necessary to give a larger amount than in intravenous injections; 5–10 c.c. m/8 or m/6 solution of sodium citrate must be introduced subcutaneously in order to produce increased peristalsis.

If the solution be introduced into the stomach or intestine a similar increase in peristalsis is brought about, but only after a considerable interval. Usually no effect is obtained until 10 to 15 minutes after the injection of the salt into the lumen of the gut. The injection may be made by piercing the wall of the intestine or stomach with a hypodermic needle, and forcing the fluid into the lumen. The quantity of the solution necessary to produce increased peristalsis is about the same as when introduced subcutaneously. The movements begin not particularly in the part of the intestine containing the solution, but simultaneously in all parts.

To any one making these experiments there can be no doubt that the increased peristalsis is the direct result of the injection of the salt. It can be readily proven in the following way: As will be shown in a later chapter, the peristalsis and secretion caused by the saline purgatives can be inhibited by the administration of calcium or magnesium chloride. If now in a rabbit in which the intestine has been set into active motion by the intravenous injection of sodium citrate, a small quantity of m/6 $CaCl_2$ be administered intravenously, all of these movements cease within a minute or two. A second injection of a slightly greater quantity of m/6 sodium citrate will overcome this action and cause active peristalsis to begin again. These actions cannot be due to anything but the solutions introduced.

It is evident also in watching the action of these salts that they produce increased peristalsis much more rapidly and powerfully when introduced intravenously than when placed in the lumen of the stomach or intestine. A much smaller dose also is required to produce this effect. They therefore cannot act because of their presence in the lumen of the gut, or because of their being subsequently secreted into the lumen. When introduced into the stomach or intestine they must first be absorbed into the blood before they can reach the muscular and glandular tissues upon which they act. They therefore act more slowly and only in larger quantities when administered in this way.

Experiments similar to the above were made with a number of salts, including sodium sulphate, fluoride, tartrate, phosphate and oxalate, barium chloride, and magnesium sulphate. It was found that intravenous and subcutaneous injections of all of these were active in producing a greater or less increase in peristalsis. Sodium sulphate acted in this respect very much as sodium citrate did. The latter, however, tended to produce muscular twitchings in the voluntary muscles, a phenomenon which will be spoken of later. Sodium sulphate on the other hand could be introduced into the blood in relatively large quantities without producing any evil effects. The action of sodium sulphate on the intestine was found to be somewhat less than that of sodium citrate; but almost constantly 2–3 c.c. m/6 Na_2SO_4 injected into the marginal vein of the ear caused a marked increase in the peristaltic movements of the intestine. I cannot at all agree with Hay and earlier writers who affirm that sodium sulphate injected intravenously produces no purgative effect. In all my experiments I have found it to have a very definite effect when introduced in this manner, and I can only attribute their results to the concentrated solutions used, or to other unfavorable conditions.

The injection of solutions of sodium fluoride produces

very active movements, although only small quantities can be administered on account of its poisonous nature.

Barium chloride is even more poisonous and only the most minute doses can be given. It is, however, by far the most powerful of all these purgative salts. Its action is extremely rapid and violent. When given intravenously it is best to mix it with about five times its volume of m/6 NaCl solution. Thus 1 c.c. of a mixture of 5 c.c. m/6 NaCl $+$ 1 c.c. m/6 $BaCl_2$ injected into the circulation causes almost immediately most violent intestinal movements. The loops contract so that they resemble white firm cords. They rise up from one another so that they seem to stand erect and the squirming, twisting movements become extremely active. The intestinal contents are hastened on and can be watched through the thin walls moving rapidly from loop to loop. The actual passage of faeces takes place in a very short time. It begins with solid faecal masses, followed quickly by semifluid faeces. The quantity passed is sometimes very considerable. As will be shown in a later chapter, the injection of $BaCl_2$ into the blood causes not only an extensive increase in the peristaltic movements, but brings about also an increase in the quantity of fluid secreted into the intestine.

The subcutaneous injection of 2–3 c.c. m/6 $BaCl_2$ produces in 5–10 minutes an effect quite similar to that described for the intravenous injection of the salt. A rabbit weighing 1,200–1,500 g. does not, however, usually recover from a dose greater than 2.5–3 c.c. m/6 $BaCl_2$ given subcutaneously, and a smaller quantity is sufficient to produce purgation. Boehm[27] gives as the lethal dose of $BaCl_2$ when given intravenously for rabbits 0.1–0.2 g., for cats 0.03–0.05 g., for dogs 0.1–0.2 g. When given subcutaneously it is 0.12–0.18 g. for rabbits and cats and 0.3 g. for dogs.

When $BaCl_2$ is taken into the stomach it is absorbed quite slowly, but its effects are similar to those described above. Active peristaltic movements and purgation result, and in many cases vomiting is seen in dogs.

It is clear from these experiments that all salts do not act equally on the intestine. Sodium chloride may be introduced in large quantities into the circulation without causing increased peristalsis or defaecation. Sodium oxalate and phosphate (Na_2HPO_4) exert only a slight action. Sodium phosphate, according to Bunge, increases the fluid in the intestine. Sodium tartrate produces quite active movements of the intestine and is considerably stronger in its action than either the oxalate or phosphate. Sodium citrate and sulphate as described above are quite constant and vigorous in their action, while barium chloride is by far the most powerful of all these saline purgatives. Sodium fluoride also acts very rapidly.

In addition to their action on the intestine, some of these salts affect the salivary gland. After the injection of $BaCl_2$ there is often so great a flow of saliva that it falls in drops from the mouth. This phenomenon is not constant, however, and seems to follow only large doses. Sodium fluoride has sometimes the same effect. I have not noticed any influence exerted by the other purgative salts upon the salivary secretion. It is further of not infrequent occurrence to have a repeated evacuation of urine after the administration of $BaCl_2$. Although this cannot be attributed to a direct increase of the secretion of urine, it is interesting to note in this connection some later experiments in which it was shown[28] that when the flow of urine in a rabbit had been well established by the injection of m/6 NaCl solution into the circulation, the addition of a minute quantity of $BaCl_2$ to the NaCl solution caused a very considerable increase in the secretion of urine from the kidney. A quantity of not more than 1/8 c.c. m/8 $BaCl_2$ must be

---

[28] MacCallum, J. B.: Journal of Exp. Zoology, Vol. I, No. 1, 1904. Preliminary Report, University of California Publications, Physiology, Vol. I, No. 10, p. 81, 1904.

given intravenously to produce this effect. If 1 c.c. m/8 $BaCl_2$ be injected intravenously at one time the flow of urine suddenly stops. This seems to be due either to a sudden constriction of the musculature of the urinary passages and pelvis of the kidney by which the lumen is cut off, or to a similar constriction of the blood vessels of the kidney. In either case the action of $BaCl_2$ in stopping the secretion is mechanical and has to do with its power of causing violent muscular contractions rather than with its capacity for increasing the secretory activity. Although there is apparently one action for $BaCl_2$ on the flow of urine when given in small doses and quite the opposite action when it is given in larger quantities, the two actions are in reality quite distinct, one being exerted on the secretory cells of the kidney and the other on the musculature of either the urinary passages or of the blood vessels of the kidney.

In addition to their action on the intestine and in some cases the kidney and salivary gland, these salts produce an interesting condition of the voluntary muscles. As mentioned above, Loeb was able to produce muscular twitchings in the muscle of a frog by immersing the muscle in solutions of these various salts. He also produced muscular twitching in a living frog by injecting sodium citrate into the dorsal lymph sacs. I have found that a subcutaneous injection of 10 c.c. m/1 sodium citrate produces in a rabbit well marked twitchings of the muscles all over the body. These are very noticeable in the gluteal region. They begin almost immediately in the neighborhood of the injection, but only after an interval of 20 to 25 minutes on the opposite side of the body. If the animal be placed on the floor it moves with a peculiar incoördinated gait. The hind legs are dragged and very little headway is made. If the rabbit be held up by the ears, the feet tremble, and if touched the legs jerk away violently and usually become rigid. There are sometimes tetanus-like contractions of the limbs, and occasionally general convulsions of greater or less severity. In one rabbit I gave daily injections of 5 c.c. m/1 sodium citrate subcutaneously throughout one month. For some time after the injections had been discontinued the hypersensitiveness seemed to persist. It seemed possible from this that a chronic state of increased irritability might be produced. No conclusion, however, can be drawn from this one experiment since the irritation caused by the repeated injections might have had some influence. It is a subject which is of interest for further experiment, on account of the similarity such a chronic condition bears to the various chronic hypersensitive conditions found in human beings.

In looking over the experiments made by various investigators on this subject it will be noticed that their results are inconstant and contradictory. This can only be the result of imperfect technique and unfavorable conditions, or of the adoption of a criterion of the action of the salt, which is uncertain. As mentioned above, the solutions used in many cases were not at all those most favorable for introduction into the blood. The very concentrated solutions used by Hay rendered the conditions obviously unfavorable. If in addition to watching for the actual passage of faeces these experimenters had observed the intestines directly the results would of necessity have been more uniform.

My own experiments have given quite uniform results, so much so that the production of increased peristalsis in rabbits by the intravenous injection of one of the saline purgatives has come to be a class experiment with the students in the medical school here. The increased secretion into the intestine produced by the same means requires greater care in protecting the loops from loss of heat and moisture. For any one to convince himself that a salt may act as a purgative when injected subcutaneously or intravenously it is only necessary to introduce a small amount of BaCl$_2$ into the blood or under the skin of a rabbit. The evacuation of large quantities of semifluid faeces and the violent intestinal movements leave no room for doubt as to the action of the salt. The fact that the intravenous and subcutaneous administration of this salt as a purgative by veterinarians is in general use should be sufficient proof.

The milder salts such as sodium citrate and sulphate must, as stated above, be given in larger quantities, and a more prolonged action is necessary.

As will be described in detail in the next chapter, the application of solutions of these salts, isosmotic with the blood, to the peritoneal surfaces of the intestine cause not only increased peristalsis and increased secretion of fluid into the intestine but also bring about an evacuation of faeces. This fact alone proves that it is not necessary to introduce the purgative salt into the stomach or intestine. The action on the intestine in this case takes place more rapidly than in any other method of administration. The solution seems to be directly absorbed through the peritoneal covering and to come into contact with the muscles and glands, and perhaps the nerves of the intestine. These tissues are immediately set into activity.

In the intravenous or subcutaneous injections of the salts it is necessary to mention a peculiarity of magnesium sulphate. This salt of course acts as a purgative because it is a sulphate and not on account of the presence of magnesium. As shown later on, magnesium chloride has an effeet quite opposite to this. In injecting MgSO$_4$ into the blood the greatest care must be taken because of its peculiarly poisonous nature when rapidly absorbed. Rabbits frequently die suddenly from an injection of a relatively small quantity. This fact has been mentioned by a number of authors, and is repeated here only as a warning against its too rapid injection, possibly in human beings.

It may be mentioned here also that Bottazzi[29] has found

---

[29] Arch. di Fisiologia, 1904, I, 413.

that the intravenous injection of an extract of the small intestine containing secretin causes not only a well marked increase in the secretion of fluid into the intestine, but also produces increased peristaltic activity. It at the same time increases the pancreatic secretion.

CHAPTER III.

The Local Application of Saline Solutions
Peritoneal Surfaces of the Intestine.

In the last chapter it has been shown that the neous and intravenous injections of solutions of saline purgatives produce a characteristic purgati and that similar injections of calcium or magues ride inhibit this action and bring the intestines to

I have found also that solutions of these salts same effect when applied directly to the peritone of the intestine. Thus if a solution of sodium sulphate,[30] for example, be poured over the intes loops which are moistened by the solution will bec within one minute. After a very short time the loops are also set in motion. These movements n tirely inhibited by pouring on the loops a soluti cium or magnesium chloride. The following des these experiments is taken directly from my pa

Strong contractions of the muscle coats took place. After a few minutes the other loops were also set in movement, so that the whole small intestine showed active peristalsis. The citrate solution was then washed off by m/6 NaCl solution, and about 3 c.c. m/6 CaCl$_2$ solution poured on the loops. The peristaltic movements were promptly suppressed, and the intestine remained quiet. By the further addition of citrate solution, the coils were set in active movement once more, and by the subsequent application of calcium chloride solution again inhibited. This was repeated many times (sixteen) and apparently might have been continued as long as the intestine remained alive.

The same results were obtained by using instead of the sodium citrate solution, a solution of barium chloride, sodium sulphate, fluoride, bromide, iodide, phosphate (Na$_3$ PO$_4$), oxalate or tartrate. Local application of solutions of any of these salts produces increased peristaltic activity. Solutions of sodium chloride have a very slight action of the same character. On the other hand, the intestinal movements are equally inhibited by calcium chloride and magnesium chloride, while strontium chloride has a similar but less powerful inhibiting action.

In testing those salts with which it was necessary to use dilutions greater than m/8, the dilution was made with a neutral fluid consisting of sodium chloride and magnesium chloride. It was found that m/6 NaCl solution increased to a very slight extent the peristaltic movements. By adding to 10 c.c. m/6 NaCl, 0.5 c.c. m/6 MgCl$_2$, a fluid was obtained which had apparently neither stimulating nor inhibiting effects. In addition to solutions made up by dilution with this neutral fluid, others were used in which the salt solutions were diluted with distilled water. Practically the same results were obtained in both cases. It was found that 1 c.c. m/320 BaCl$_2$ solution applied locally to the intestine is sufficient to cause strong peristaltic movements in a rabbit. This quantity contains about 0.00076 gm. barium

chloride. In the case of sodium citrate, the concentra
must be considerably greater. No solution of this salt 1
dilute than m/80 is active in a rabbit. Of all the purge
salts, barium chloride is by far the most powerful.
drop of m/8 $BaCl_2$ be placed on the serous surface o:
intestinal loop, or if a small area be moistened with
solution by means of a camel's hair brush, the muscle
neath the moistened area will almost immediately cont
so that a ring-like constriction of the intestine is for1
This often is so sharply marked that it suggests the e
produced by tying a ligature around the intestine. '
constriction remains for a few moments, and then gradu
moves along the loop in the direction of the normal p
talsis. If the solution be injected into the muscle of
intestine at any point with a hypodermic needle, a sin
sharp constriction takes place. If also a few drops be
jected directly into a branch of the superior mesent
artery, all that part of the loop supplied by the arte
branch will contract violently. These statements are '
also in the case of sodium citrate, fluoride, sulphate, (
he action of these salts, however, is less powerful.

It must be added here also that the actual passag
faeces may be produced within an hour by the applica
of the purgative salts to the serous surfaces of the intest
This takes place most quickly with barium chloride. 1
possible to observe directly through the semi-transpa:
walls of the intestine the rapid passage of faecal ma
from one loop to another.

The intestines of the rabbit are apparently much n
sensitive to the action of sodium citrate and sulphate t
are those of the dog or cat. Barium chloride, on the
rary, acts with equal strength in all these animals. 1
rabbit, the intestines are always set in active perist
movement by contact with m/8 sodium citrate solution;
even much more dilute solutions are, as a rule, effective.
cat, however, it was found that an m/8 solution of sod

citrate has practically no effect, while a 5/8m solution sets the intestine in active motion. In a dog also m/8 sodium citrate solution is usually ineffective. Similarly an m/8 sodium sulphate solution is inactive in a dog while an m/2 solution of the same salt starts up distinct peristalsis. In the cat and dog also the peristalsis may be inhibited by calcium or magnesium chloride, as shown in the following experiments. The intestines of a cat were exposed in the usual manner, and an m/8 solution of sodium citrate was applied to the serous surface of the loops. There was no increased movement. There were then poured on the loops a few cubic centimetres of a mixture of 5 c.c. 5/8m sodium citrate and 5 c.c. 5/8m $CaCl_2$. The loops remained motionless. After waiting a considerable time (15 minutes), a 5/8m solution of sodium citrate alone was poured on the intestine. Almost immediately they became very active; and the peristalsis continued until calcium chloride was again applied. The loops then came to a standstill. The difference in susceptibility to the action of citrate which exists between rabbits on the one hand, and dogs and cats on the other, may be in some way connected with their being herbivorous and carnivorous animals respectively.

The action of the sodium citrate, sulphate, fluoride, etc., when applied locally, may be inhibited by the administration of an approximately equal quantity of calcium or magnesium chloride of the same concentration. The counteraction of the effect of barium chloride, however, requires a much greater concentration of calcium. Using equal quantities of the two salts, the action of the barium is usually not inhibited, a fact which I have previously stated. With greater concentrations of the calcium chloride, the antagonistic action, however, is clear. This is shown in the following experiment: Applied locally to the intestine of a rabbit 1 c.c. m/320 $BaCl_2$ solution caused active peristaltic movements. The application of 1 c.c. m/320 $CaCl_2$ solution exercised no inhibiting effect whatever. The same quantity of m/40 $CaCl_2$ was then poured on the loops, and a slight but distinct quieting of the loops took place. The addition of 1 c.c. m/6 $CaCl_2$ caused the loops to become entirely motionless. After waiting a considerable time, 1 c.c. m/8 $BaCl_2$ was poured on the intestine. Immediately violent peristaltic movements took place. Several c.c. m/6 $CaCl_2$ exercised practically no inhibiting influence; while 2 c.c. 5/8m $CaCl_2$ solution suppressed the movements entirely for a short time.

The question concerning the exact seat of action of the purgative salts remains still unanswered. Whether, upon being absorbed into the blood, they act on the central nervous system is not known. There is no evidence to show that this is the case. It seems certain, on the other hand, from the experiments here described, that they undoubtedly have a peripheral action either on the peripheral nervous mechanism or on the muscle cells themselves. It is impossible to prove that there is no action on the central nervous system, and at present it seems impossible to prove whether the peripheral action is directly on the nerves or on the muscles. The existence in the walls of the intestine of the ganglionic plexuses of Auerbach and Meissner must be taken into consideration; and with the methods available there seems to be no way of distinguishing the action on these plexuses and the direct action on the muscle cells. The ultimate effect is on the muscles and glands; and the fact that an entirely local ring-shaped constriction can be brought about by the local application of a drop of one of the salt solutions to the surface of the intestine would seem to indicate that only a small group of the circular muscle fibres themselves is affected. The fact that the nerve plexuses form a continuous network, and are intimately related in their various parts, would suggest that the occurrence of an action on these plexuses confined to so small an area is improbable. The discussion of the exact location of the action is, however, of relatively little importance, as compared with the main facts shown by these experiments, namely, that *it is possible to produce, by the local application of a purgative salt to the serous surface of the intestine, a striking increase in peristalsis, and to suppress these movements by a similar application of solutions of calcium, magnesium, or strontium chloride.*

These experiments also seem to decide the question as to whether the salt solutions act after being absorbed into the blood or only when placed in the intestine. According to Hay[32] and others, the salt which is absorbed into the circulation has no effect and the only action is produced by that which remains in the intestine. This is obviously not true since the solutions act much more rapidly and more powerfully when applied to the outside of the intestine, *i.e.,* to the peritoneal surface. No action is observed until after an interval of 10 to 15 minutes after the salt solution is placed in the lumen of the intestine, while application of the same solution to the peritoneal surface causes movements of the intestine within one minute.

---

[32] *Loc. cit.*

CHAPTER IV.

'roduction of Increased Secretion of Fluid
ı the Intestine by the Saline Purgatives.

f the most characteristic things to be observed in
. is the presence of a greater quantity of fluid in
. This varies in degree with the different drugs,
vith the mild laxatives the faeces become less solid.
stronger purgatives they become quite fluid.

earliest attempts to explain the nature of pur-
ere has been the question as to the origin of this
ith the discovery of the property of osmosis in
w life was given to this inquiry, and Poiseuille[33]
the theory that the purgative effect of salts was
ely to their endosmotic power, the increased fluid
ices being caused by the extraction of fluid from
is by the osmotic power of the salt. The same
held by Liebig,[34] whose name is commonly asso-
h the hypothesis. Rabuteau[35] later on supported
and claimed as proof of it the fact that he was
ı produce purgation by the intravenous injec-
large quantities of sodium sulphate. He even
ıt this injection caused constipation, and he con-
at since sodium sulphate purges when given by
are must be caused a flow of fluid towards the salt

—
:ch. expériment. sur les mouvements des liquides dans les
ıtits diamètres, Paris, 1828. Comptes rendus t. 19, 1844.
n Hay.
lie Saftbewegung, 1848.
on Médicale, 1871, Nos. 50 et 52. Gaz. Méd. de Paris, 1879.

in both cases. This osmosis theory was attacked by Claude Bernard,[36] who pointed out that if the purgative action of salts were due to their osmotic power, sugar must also be a strong purgative. He found further that, contrary to what Rabuteau stated, intravenous injections of sodium sulphate do cause purgation and bring it about more rapidly and powerfully than when the salt is taken by mouth. It was further shown by Aubert[37] that the purgative effect of various salts is not at all proportional to their endosmotic power nor to their concentration. Headland,[38] assuming without experiment that purgative salts act when introduced into the circulation, advanced the hypothesis that when they are given by mouth they are first absorbed into the blood and are later excreted by the intestine. In thus passing through the intestine he supposed that they stimulated the glands to secrete. Brieger,[39] using the method introduced by Colin and Moreau, obtained what he considered an increased secretion into the intestine. Isolating a loop of the intestine, he introduced into it a strong solution of $MgSO_4$. The loop became in a short time filled with a clear yellow alkaline fluid. This he believed was due partly to the water attracting power of the salt, and partly to the production of a real secretion. Vulpian[40] believed that the fluid was due to an inflammatory irritation. Hay[41] made experiments similar to those of Brieger, and found that the introduction into a loop of 10% Na_2SO_4 caused a considerable increase in the secretion, although no secretion was obtained by a 1–5% solution. Schmiedeberg[42] explained the presence of a greater quantity of fluid in the stools following the administration of the purgative by the supposition that the

---

[36] Leçons sur les effets des substances toxiques et médicamenteuses, Paris, 1857.
[37] Zeitsch. f. Rationelle Medicin, Bd. 1, 1851.
[38] Action of Medicines, 1857.
[39] Archiv f. exp. Path. u. Pharm., Bd. VIII, 1878, S. 355.
[40] Gazette Médicale, 1873.
[41] Journal of Physiology, Vol. XVI, 1882.
[42] Arzneimittellehre, Leipzig, 1883.

purgative salts on reaching the large intestine p
absorption of water. He states that these salts
selves absorbed with difficulty and hence reach
part of the intestine unchanged. A similar hy
advanced by Wallace and Cushny.[43] They state
absorption of fluid was inhibited especially by
which form insoluble compounds with calciu
authors, however, did not take into account the
of the secretion of fluid into the intestine being in
these salts. Hence their method of determining
ence in absorption of the various solutions is op
cism, since it will be shown in this chapter that s
all of these purgative salts cause a very definite
the intestinal fluid. The absorption of fluid may
diminished by these salts, but it is difficult to
experiments of Wallace and Cushny how much o
remaining in the loops is due to inhibited absor
how much has been actually secreted by the inte

The experiments of Brieger[44] and Hay[45] in t
tion of increased secretion are quite unsatisfact
count of the great concentration of the solut
Their results may well be ascribed to the local
effect of the strong solution, since they did not
increased secretion with weaker solutions.

As stated above in a previous section, I ha
large number of experiments to determine whet
an increased secretion is actually caused by the s
atives, and have found by measurements that wi

neons injection of 4–5 c.c. 1% morphine hydrochlorate. The rabbits were not full grown, their average weight being not more than 1,200 g. The same amount of morphine was given also to the dogs, and was supplemented by ether. The abdominal cavity was opened and a loop of considerable length tied off with ligatures. In the rabbit the upper part of the small intestine was selected and the upper ligature placed just below the entrance of the common bile duct. The second ligature was tied 25 to 30 cm. lower down. At the lower end of the loop a large mouthed cannula was inserted from which the fluid could be drained by gently lifting the successive parts of the loop, a process made more easy by placing the animal board at a considerable angle with the table. All of this was done as rapidly as possible, so that the loops would be exposed as little as possible to the air. After the loop had been emptied of what it contained in this way, the intestines were covered over with filter paper soaked in warm m/6 NaCl solution, and this again covered with a towel wet with warm water, and over it all a woolen cloth. In this way the loops were protected fairly well from drying and loss of heat. The contact with the wet filter paper did not seem in any way to affect the intestine. Other experiments were made with the filter paper raised from the intestine by a wire tent. I found that if these precautions against loss of heat and drying were neglected the secretion did not take place. The greatest care must be exercised in this respect since the slightest cooling seems to inhibit the secretory activity of the intestine.

The loop which had thus been emptied and returned to moist warm surroundings was left 10 minutes and the normal secretion allowed to collect, and at the end of that period the loop was again emptied with as little exposure as possible and the fluid measured. The cannula was then clamped off and the secretion allowed to gather for a second 10 minutes. This again was drawn off and measured. The quantity secreted was usually fairly constant and quite small, the manipulation undoubtedly increasing it somewhat. When the normal secretion was obtained the purgative salt in an isotonic solution was administered either subcutaneously, intravenously, or locally. The secretion was again allowed to collect, and was drained off and measured after 10 minutes. This was repeated several times and the amounts compared with what was taken as the normal secretion. When the solution was applied locally, a method which is perhaps the most satisfactory, it was allowed to drop on the loops from a pipette, care being taken to have it at body temperature and as nearly as possible isosmotic with the blood. In each case special care was taken to have no interval between the emptying of the loop and the beginning of the succeeding period of 10 minutes. In other words, the loop was always entirely empty at the beginning of each period.

The results of a few of these experiments may be seen in the following reports:—

1. Rabbit.   Loop 30 cm. long, upper part of small intestine.
 Loop contained in beginning[47] .... 5.0 c.c.
 Fluid removed after 1st 10 minutes .... 0.2 c.c.
 Fluid removed after 2d 10 minutes .... 0.5 c.c.
  2 c.c. m/8 BaCl$_2$ injected subcutaneously.
 Fluid removed after 1st 10 minutes following injection 4.0 c.c.
 Fluid removed after 2d 10 minutes following injection 3.4 c.c.
 Fluid removed after 3d 10 minutes following injection 3.0 c.c.

In this rabbit the increased secretion of fluid was accompanied by extremely active peristaltic movements. The faeces could be seen passing along the loops of the lower part of the intestine with great rapidity. Within 30 minutes after the administration of the salt, the passage of faeces to the outside began. This continued for some time,

---

[47] In all these experiments there was no interval beteen the emptying of the loop and the beginning of the 10-minute period which followed. The injections were made as rapidly as possible, and in no case occupied more than a minute.

34

the faeces becoming constantly softer, until finally they were almost entirely unformed.

As shown by this experiment, and also by the following ones, the action of barium chloride persists for a considerable length of time. The action of sodium citrate is more transitory.

2. Rabbit. Loop 25 cm. long.
    Loop contained in beginning .... 3.0 c.c. fluid deeply bile stained
    After 1st 10 minutes.... 1.0 c.c. fluid deeply bile stained
    After 2d 10 minutes.... 0.8 c.c. fluid somewhat lighter in color
Injected 2 c.c. m/8 BaCl$_2$ solution subcutaneously.
    After 1st 10 min. following injection ...... 2.5 c.c. fluid light yellow
    After 2d 10 min. following injection ...... 1.6 c.c. fluid very light yellow
    After 3d 10 min. following injection ...... 1.8 c.c. fluid almost colorless
    After 4th 10 min. following injection ...... 1.6 c.c. fluid quite colorless
    After 5th 10 min. following injection ...... 1.0 c.c. fluid quite colorless
3. Rabbit. Loop 32 cm. long.
    Loop contained in beginning .... 6.0 c.c.
    After 1st 10 minutes .... 0.4 c.c.
    After 2d 10 minutes .... 0.1 c.c.
    After 3d 10 minutes .... 0.4 c.c.
Poured 5 c.c. m/8 sodium citrate on loop.
    After 1st 10 minutes .... 6.2 c.c.
    After 2d 10 minutes .... 2.0 c.c.
4. Dog. Loop 35 cm. long,
    Loop contained no fluid, *i.e.*, none could be drained off.
    After 1st 10 minutes .... 0.0 c.c.
    After 2d 10 minutes .... 0.0 c.c.
    After 3d 10 minutes .... 0.0 c.c.
Poured 3 c.c. m/8 BaCl$_2$ on loop.
    After 1st 20 minutes .... 8.0 c.c.
    After 2d 20 minutes .... 0.6 c.c.
Poured 1½ c.c. m/8 BaCl$_2$ on loop just enough to moisten it.
    After 1st 20 minutes .... 3.2 c.c.
    After 2d 20 minutes .... 2.5 c.c.

From these experiments, in which every precaution was taken, it seems certain that a definite increase in the secretion of fluid into the intestine follows the administration of barium chloride, and sodium citrate, the former of which is a saline purgative of a more powerful type, while the latter is among the milder purgative salts. It is of especial interest that these salts do not produce the increase of fluid on account of an irritating effect on the mucous membrane of the intestine. The action takes place, as shown in the experiments, when they are introduced subcutaneously or directly applied to the peritoneal surface of the intestine. Further, the solutions were practically isosmotic with the blood, and for this reason and from the fact that they were applied to the peritoneal surface of the intestine the osmotic pressure of the solution could play no part in causing fluid to enter the lumen of the gut. Also it is obvious that any possible effect which the purgatives may have in delaying absorption from the intestine (Wallace and Cushny) could have nothing to do with the production of this increased amount of fluid in the loops experimented with. The fluid produced is clear and either colorless or slightly yellow. It has an alkaline reaction and is apparently quite similar to the normal intestinal secretion. I have made no experiments to determine its powers of digesting and have no data concerning this point. There are no signs of its being of an inflammatory nature.

Thinking that the manipulation of the intestine and the tying off of loops might influence the results, I estimated from the examination of a large number of rabbits of the same size (about 1,200 g. in weight) the quantity of fluid which is normally found in the small intestine. It was found that there was hardly ever more than 10 c.c., and usually only 5 or 6 c.c. of fluid in addition to a small amount of semifluid food material. To a rabbit in which the intestines seemed almost empty, a small dose of barium chloride was given locally by pouring an m/8 solution on the loops. The characteristic effect of the barium followed, and after one hour the small intestine was tied off by ligatures and removed. It was found to contain 22 c.c. of a clear yellowish fluid. In a second rabbit which received the same treatment 34 c.c. of a similar fluid were found in the small intestine.

As will be shown in a later chapter, a secretion of fluid into the lumen of isolated loops of intestine removed from the body may be produced by immersing the loops, with their ends tied, in solutions of various saline purgatives. In m/8 solutions of NaCl, Na_2SO_4, and sodium citrate no secretion was obtained in these loops. In m/2 solution of these salts, however, a distinct measurable quantity was regularly produced; m/8 solutions of NaF brought about a secretion, and in all solutions containing $BaCl_2$ a distinct secretion of fluid was obtained. This will be described in detail later on.

As stated above, Bottazzi has found that an extract of the small intestine, which increases the secretion of pancreatic juice, is capable also when injected intravenously of increasing not only the secretory activity of the intestine, but also its peristalsis.

As stated in detail in another chapter, the secretion of fluid into the intestine, as well as the peristaltic movements, is inhibited by the administration of calcium or magnesium chloride. This is illustrated by the following experiments :—

1. Rabbit. Loop 23 cm. long.

Loop contained in beginning .... 0.9 c.c.
Fluid secreted during 1st 10 minutes .... 0.7 c.c.
Fluid secreted during 2d 10 minutes .... 0.6 c.c.
2 c.c. m/8 $CaCl_2$ applied locally.
Fluid secreted during 1st 10 minutes .... 0.15 c.c.
Fluid secreted during 2d 10 minutes .... 0.0 c.c.
Fluid secreted during 3d 10 minutes .... 0.0 c.c.
4 c.c. m/8 sodium citrate applied locally.
Fluid secreted during 1st 10 minutes .... 0.4 c.c.
Fluid secreted during 2d 10 minutes .... 0.2 c.c.

2. Rabbit. Loop 25 cm. long.
    Loop contained in beginning .... 2.0 c.c.
    Fluid secreted during 1st 10 minutes .... 0.8 c.c.
    Fluid secreted during 2d 10 minutes .... 0.4 c.c.
    2 c.c. m/8 CaCl$_2$ applied locally to serous surface.
    Fluid secreted during 1st 10 minutes following appli-
        cation .... 0.0 c.c.
    Fluid secreted during 2d 10 minutes following appli-
        cation .... 0.0 c.c.
    4 c.c. m/8 sodium citrate applied locally.
    Fluid secreted during 1st 10 minutes .... 0.6 c.c.
3. Rabbit. Loop 22 cm. long.
    Loop contained in beginning .... 2.4 c.c.
    Fluid secreted during 1st 10 minutes .... 1.2 c.c.
    Fluid secreted during 2d 10 minutes .... 1.15 c.c.
    3 c.c. m/8 MgCl$_2$ applied locally to serous surface.
    Fluid secreted during 1st 10 minutes following appli-
        cation .... 0.0 c.c.
    Fluid secreted during 2d 10 minutes following appli-
        cation .... 0.0 c.c.
    Fluid secreted during 3d 10 minutes following appli-
        cation .... 0.2 c.c.

Although in these experiments the quantity of fluid secreted is small, there is a definite cessation of this excretion following the application of calcium or magnesium chloride. The subsequent administration of sodium citrate in each case causes the secretion to recommence.

CHAPTER V.

The Inhibiting Action of Calcium and Magnesium on the Movements and Secretion of the Intestine.

It was first observed by Ringer[48] that the unfavorable effect produced by pure NaCl solution could be lessened by adding other salts, notably calcium and potassium. From this observation there was made the so-called Ringer's solution, which contains Na, K, and Ca in proportions which render the solution relatively neutral and innocuous towards the living tissues.

Howell,[49] working with the heart of the terrapin in various mixtures of Na, K, and Ca chloride, emphasized the importance of calcium in the medium in which the heart beat. He concluded from his experiments that the sodium chloride was mainly instrumental in establishing and maintaining the proper osmotic conditions, while calcium was the main factor in initiating and maintaining the beat of the heart. To quote from his articles:—"The stimulus that leads to a heart contraction is dependent upon the presence of calcium compounds in the liquids of the heart; but for rhythmic contractions and relaxations a certain proportion of potassium compounds is necessary." "The sodium chloride seems to be essential only in preserving the osmotic relations between the tissues and the surrounding liquid." Similar conclusions were arrived at by Green.[50]

[48] Journal of Physiology, Vols. 4, 5, 6, 8, 16, 17, and 18, 1883-1895.
[49] Amer. Journ. Physiol., Vol. 2, 1898, p. 47.
[50] Amer. Journ. Physiol., Vol. 2, 1898, p. 82.

Loeb,[51] working with Gonionemus, and with the striated muscles of the frog, arrived at conclusions which are in some respects entirely opposed to those of Howell. What Loeb spoke of as the toxic effects of sodium chloride was emphasized by this work. This was especially shown in the case of Fundulus eggs which, though freshly fertilized, cannot develop in pure NaCl solution, although they develop in sea-water or in distilled water. In this case the addition of a small quantity of calcium chloride to the NaCl rendered development possible. According to Loeb, the Ca exerted an antitoxic effect and neutralized the injurious action of the NaCl. Similarly it was found that the apex of the heart contracts rhythmically in a pure NaCl solution, but soon came to a standstill. The addition of a small amount of calcium is sufficient to cause the contractions to persist for a long time. This again was referred to the toxic and antitoxic effects of the salts. From these and similar experiments arose the conception of "physiologically balanced solutions" in which the toxic effect of each substance in the solution is exactly counteracted by the antitoxic effect of some other substance in the same solution.

Other experiments by Loeb showed that if the voluntary muscle of a frog be immersed in a pure NaCl solution, rhythmical twitchings appear which continue for many hours, or even for days. If, however, a small quantity of $CaCl_2$ be added to the NaCl solution the twitchings cease, although the muscle remains alive in this mixture longer than it does in pure NaCl. Similar results were obtained with solutions of the sodium salts which precipitate calcium, fluoride, oxalate, carbonate, phosphate, etc. In all of these solutions twitchings developed in the muscle. Magnesium and strontium act like calcium in inhibiting the muscular twitchings produced by sodium salts. These experiments led Loeb to the conclusion that the presence of

[51] Festschrift f. Fick, 1899. Chicago Decennial Publications, 1902, and Pflüger's Archiv, Bd. 91, S. 248, 1902. Amer. Journ. Physiol., Vol. 5, 1901.

calcium in the body keeps the voluntary muscles from constantly twitching or beating rhythmically in the way the heart does. Calcium, magnesium, and strontium seemed to have a definite inhibitory action on the muscular contractions.

Loeb further showed that the center of a jellyfish (Gonionemus), which when isolated from the margin will not contract in sea-water, will beat rhythmically if placed in pure NaCl solution. If a quantity of $CaCl_2$ or $Ca(NO_3)_2$ be added to the NaCl solution the contractions are inhibited. Magnesium and strontium behave in this respect like calcium. If also a sufficient quantity of a calcium precipitating solution (sodium fluoride, phosphate, etc.) be added to sea-water in which the center will not beat, rhythmical contractions soon appear, due apparently to the removal of the calcium from the sea-water and the tissue. In these experiments, as in those with voluntary muscles, calcium magnesium and strontium have apparently an inhibiting action on muscular contractions.

Loeb has recently made experiments on a jellyfish of the Pacific (Polyorchis) with results which are somewhat different from those described for voluntary muscles and Gonionemus. He found that the normal swimming movements of the uninjured animal could not occur in solutions which did not contain some proportion of magnesium, and the presence of magnesium in the sea-water seemed to be the stimulus for the apparently spontaneous movements of the animal. Calcium and potassium were found to oppose this action of magnesium. Further with the isolated center of Polyorchis, which will not beat in pure sugar solution or in sea-water, it was found that the addition of $CaCl_2$, $SrCl_2$, or $BaCl_2$ to either solution caused contractions to appear. Magnesium chloride did not produce this effect. In pure NaCl solution also the isolated center will not beat, or beats only after a long time, while the addition of $CaCl_2$ to the NaCl causes it to beat at once.

Lingle[52] made experiments with the ventricle of the tortoise heart, which was able to beat for only a short time in pure NaCl solutions. When a small amount of $CaCl_2$ is added, however, the heart may continue to beat for a long period. Lingle explained this by the assumption that NaCl is a poison and that calcium acts in an antitoxic way, a suggestion already offered by Loeb.

Loeb's experiments on the inhibition of muscular twitchings in voluntary muscles by calcium and magnesium, as well as the similar results he obtained with the isolated center of Gonionemus, led me to test the action of these two substances on the rhythmical movements of the mammalian intestine. It was found that not only the normal movements of the intestine, but also those produced by the saline purgatives such as sodium citrate, sulphate, tartrate, etc., could be very definitely inhibited by the administration of calcium or magnesium chloride. This was the case when these latter substances were given in any way either intravenously, subcutaneously, or applied directly to the serous surfaces of the intestine. The following experiments will illustrate this inhibitory action.

A rabbit was anaesthetized by a subcutaneous injection of 4-5 c.c. 1% morphine solution. The intestines were then carefully exposed and protected in every way from loss of heat and moisture. The method suggested by van Braam-Houckgeest[53] of opening the abdomen under the surface of sodium chloride solution is perhaps the most perfect. A small quantity of m/6 sodium citrate solution (for a rabbit weighing 1,200 g. 2-3 c.c. is sufficient) was injected into a vein of the ear. The intestines almost immediately began to move actively. There was then injected 3-4 c.c. m/6 $CaCl_2$ solution. The intestines within 2 or 3 minutes came entirely to rest and remained perfectly quiet. A second injection of a somewhat greater quantity of sodium citrate caused them to again become active.

---

[52] Amer. Journ. Physiol., Vol. 4, p. 265, 1900; Vol. 8, p. 75, 1902.
[53] Pflüger's Archiv, Bd. 6, 1872; and Bd. 8, 1874.

A still more striking experiment may be made by exposing the intestines and pouring a small quantity of sodium citrate solution on their peritoneal surfaces. Immediately they become extremely active. If now they be washed off with a little NaCl solution and a few c.c. of a solution of calcium chloride be poured on them they will come to rest at once. These solutions must be at body temperature and isotonic with the blood. If the loops which have been quieted by CaCl$_2$ are again moistened with the citrate solution they will be set into motion as before, and a subsequent application of CaCl$_2$ will again cause all movement to cease. This may be continued almost indefinitely. I have set the same loops in motion and stopped them by these solutions as many as sixteen times in succession.

Magnesium chloride acts in this respect like calcium chloride, and a similar but slighter action is possessed by strontium chloride. Magnesium sulphate has a purgative action just as many other sulphates have. Magnesium citrate also acts in the same way as other citrates. The action of the magnesium in these cases seems to be subordinate.

In addition to the inhibitory action of calcium and magnesium on the peristaltic movements of the intestine, these substances also suppress the secretion of fluid into the intestine. This is shown in the previous chapter (IV), where tables are given to show the course of the experiments. According to these experiments, the normal rate of secretion in an isolated loop was measured. The quantity of fluid secreted was small, but the application of CaCl$_2$ or MgCl$_2$ to the serous surface of the loop stopped the secretion entirely. The subsequent application of sodium citrate caused it to flow again.

In its counteraction of the effect of saline purgatives, calcium behaves in the same way. The increased peristalsis or secretion caused by sodium citrate, sulphate, etc., is entirely suppressed by the administration of calcium or magnesium chloride. This is not true to the same extent of those activities produced by barium chloride. $CaCl_2$ as far as I have been able to determine only partially counteracts the effect of $BaCl_2$. That an antagonism does exist cannot be doubted, but the violent peristaltic movements brought about by $BaCl_2$ cannot be fully suppressed by $CaCl_2$ or $MgCl_2$. As mentioned above, $BaCl_2$ in extremely small doses causes an increased flow of urine.[54] This can be partially inhibited by $CaCl_2$. With slightly larger doses of barium, the flow of urine often ceases abruptly, due probably to the contraction of the musculature of the urinary passages, or possibly to a contraction of the blood vessels of the kidney. This condition is relieved by the administration of $CaCl_2$, that is, the calcium merely counteracts the effect of the barium on the musculature of the urinary passages or blood vessels, whichever it may be.

Experiments have recently been made to test the effect of adding calcium salts to barium chloride and feeding the two mixed with some edible substance to mice. $BaCl_2$ is a common poison to employ for mice and rats. It was found that the mice eating food containing barium carbonate alone died, while those eating the mixture of calcium carbonate and barium carbonate in the food were unharmed.[55]

When loops of the intestine are entirely removed from the body and placed in sodium chloride solution, active movements begin, as will be described in detail in a later chapter. These movements continue 40 to 45 minutes or longer if the proper conditions of temperature, etc., are preserved. If, however, $CaCl_2$ be added to this solution the movements are inhibited. Also loops placed in pure $m/6$ $CaCl_2$ solution lie perfectly quiet.

A peculiar action of calcium which will be described in detail later on is shown in the following experiments: A loop of rabbit's intestine was removed from the body and

[54] MacCallum, J. B.: Journal exp. Zoology, No. 1, 1905.
[55] Stover, F. H.: Bulletin of Bussey Institution, Vol. II, Part IV, 1884.

placed in a solution of m/6 LiCl. After moving rhythmically for about 15 seconds the loop came to rest. A loop similarly placed in m/6 CaCl$_2$ solution showed no movements. In a mixture, however, of 50 c.c. m/6 LiCl + 5 c.c. m/6 CaCl$_2$ the initial movements seen in the pure LiCl solution were absent and the loop remained quiet for 10–15 minutes. Then sudden sharp constrictions appear in the loop, followed by violent contractions of the whole loop. The loop twists and coils upon itself and continues to move in this extremely active manner for 30–45 minutes or longer. The control loops in pure LiCl and pure CaCl$_2$ remain motionless during all this time.

A similar phenomenon occurs with a mixture of NaCl and CaCl$_2$. In NaCl, however, the initial movements are much more conspicuous and may continue for an hour. These are inhibited in the mixture of NaCl and CaCl$_2$, and after 10–15 minutes movements of an entirely different character appear, resembling those described for mixtures of LiCl and CaCl$_2$. Sharp constrictions and violent twistings persist for 30 or 40 minutes.

These peculiar contractions do not occur in mixtures of LiCl and NaCl, nor in mixtures of CaCl$_2$ and MgCl$_2$.

In addition to their action on the intestine, calcium and magnesium have a very definite action on other organs of the body, more especially the kidney. It was found[56] that both calcium and magnesium chlorides inhibit the flow of urine. This is shown in the following tables taken from the paper referred to.

---

[56] MacCallum, J. B.: Journal Exp. Zoology, Vol. I, No. 1, 1904.

Rabbit—cannula placed in bladder. No urine flowed in the first or second periods of 10 minutes before the NaCl solution was injected.

Time	Salts other than NaCl injected	m/6 NaCl injected in c.c.	Urine in c.c.
10:10	....	10	......
10:15		10	......
10:20		5	0.5
10:40		10	0.8
11:00		10	0.5
11:20		5	1.0
11:40	....	10	2.8
12:00	....	10	6.0
12:00	5 c.c. m/6 CaCl$_2$ intravenously		
12:05	5 c.c. 5m/6 CaCl$_2$ subcutaneously		
12:20	....	5	0.2
12:40	....	10	1.8
1:00	....	10	0.8
1:00	5 c.c. m/6 sodium citrate intravenously		
1:20	....	10	2.2
1:40		5	3.6

In this case, although the flow of urine was considerably increased by the injection of NaCl solution, and although the injection was continued, the introduction of CaCl$_2$ caused the flow to almost cease. This action was quite constant and was obtained in a large number of experiments. MgCl$_2$ has a similar but less powerful effect. The action of the CaCl$_2$ is temporary and wears off after a little time, as shown in the following table taken from the same paper. It represents only the latter half of the experiment, the regular injection of 2 c.c. NaCl solution per minute gradually increasing the rate of flow as shown, until the quantity of fluid excreted almost equals that injected.

Rabbit—cannula in bladder—injections intravenous.

Time	Salts other than NaCl injected	m/6 NaCl injected in c.c.	Urine in c.c.
9:25	....	......	......
11:40	....	150	64.5
11:45		10	6.6
11:50		10	5.6
11:55		10	6.2
12:00	....	10	7.4
12:05	....	10	9.5
12:05	5 c.c. m/6 CaCl$_2$		
12:10	....	5	2.2
12:15		10	0.8
12:20		10	1.2
12:25		10	1.6
12:30		10	2.8
12:35		8	3.0
12:40		5	4.5
12:45		0	4.8
12:50	....	0	5.1
12:55	....	0	6.2

It was found in another series of experiments[57] that the haemoglobinuria caused by saponin and by quillain, which is a dried extract of Quillaja bark, may be inhibited by calcium chloride. The intravenous injection of 2 c.c. $\frac{1}{4}\%$ quillain always produced haemoglobinuria in a rabbit weighing about 1,200 g. If the dilution of the quillain were made with m/6 CaCl$_2$ instead of water, e.g., 2 c.c. 1% quillain + 6 c.c. m/6 CaCl$_2$ and 2 c.c. of this injected intravenously, no haemoglobinuria resulted, although the concentration of the quillain was the same in both cases. The CaCl$_2$ does not stop the excretion of the haemoglobin by the kidneys, for if the saponin or quillain be given first and the haemoglobinuria established, the subsequent injection of CaCl$_2$ does not stop the excretion of haemoglobin. This is explained by a large number of experiments in which it was shown that the haemolysis caused by saponin, quillain, or digitalin is particularly inhibited by calcium chloride and magnesium chloride. This can be seen in the following

[57] MacCallum, J. B.: University of California Publications, Physiology, Vol. II, 1905, p. 93.

in which defibrinated rabbit's blood is used, and the
ts of CaCl$_2$ and MgCl$_2$ are compared with that of NaCl

1 c.c. blood 5 c.c. m/6 NaCl 3 drops 0.5% saponin	1 c.c. blood 5 c.c. m/6 MgCl$_2$ 3 drops 0.5% saponin	1 c.c. blood 5 c.c. m/6 CaCl$_2$ 3 drops 0.5% saponin
change of color	no change	no change
almost transparent	no change	no change
· laking almost complete	no change	no change
laking complete	no change	no change
laking complete	corpuscles settled to bottom; supernatant fluid colored; mixture quite opaque on shaking	same as MgCl$_2$ mixture

t is of considerable interest to note that these sub-
:es, saponin, quillain, and digitalin, act not only as
iolytics, but also as diuretics. This was shown in a
ber of experiments.[58] As shown in the following table,
njection of a very small quantity of saponin produces
tinct increase in the quantity of urine excreted.

Time	m/6 NaCl injected intravenously	Urine
10:15		
10:20	10 c.c.	2 c.c.
10:25	20 c.c.	4 c.c.
10:30	20 c.c.	6 c.c.
10:35	10 c.c.	7.5 c.c.
10:40	10 c.c.	8.0 c.c.
10:45	10 c.c.	8.2 c.c.
10:50	10 c.c.	7.9 c.c.
10:56	Injected 2 c.c. 1/20% saponin in m/6 NaCl	
11:00	10 c.c.	10.5 c.c.
11:05	10 c.c.	11.0 c.c.
11:10	10 c.c.	11.0 c.c.
11:15	10 c.c.	11.0 c.c.
11:16	Injected 1 c.c. 1/20% saponin	
11:20	10 c.c.	12.2 c.c.
11:25	10 c.c.	13.2 c.c.
11:30	10 c.c.	12.0 c.c.
11:35	10 c.c.	12.5 c.c.

MacCallum, J. B.: *Loc. cit.*

It is possible that it is by no means a coincidence that these substances which are powerful haemolytics act also as diuretics; and that $CaCl_2$ and $MgCl_2$, which inhibit the secretion of urine, also to some extent inhibit the haemolytic action. It is difficult to say by what process the haemoglobin is liberated from the red blood corpuscle, as indeed it is difficult to state definitely how fluid passes from the blood into the urine. It is sufficient to call attention to the fact that the liberation of haemoglobin and the flow of urine may be to some extent controlled by the same conditions. If the haemolytics such as saponin cause haemolysis by increasing the permeability of the membranes of the red blood corpuscles, it seems possible that the diuretic effect of these substances may be due to a similar process in the kidney. If this be true, changes in permeability must play an important part in the action of these diuretics. And it is not impossible that the inhibition of the haemolytic action of saponin, etc., as well as the inhibition of the flow of urine by $CaCl_2$ and $MgCl_2$, may be due to a decreased permeability of the red blood corpuscle on the one hand, and of the kidney cells on the other.

With these numerous experiments with calcium and magnesium it is still impossible to make a general statement as to the nature of their action. Since the chemical conditions existing in the tissues of animals and of various parts of animals are largely a matter of conjecture, we cannot predict how these substances will act; nor can we say that because calcium, for example, has a certain action in one animal or on one organ it will necessarily have the same action in other animals or in other organs.

In the experiments on the rabbit's intestine, however, calcium and magnesium have been shown to have an action which can only be described as inhibitory. In an animal as highly organized as the rabbit, the intestine is an extremely complex organ; it is not only a muscular and a glandular organ, but contains a complicated nervous mechanism peculiar to itself which is entirely inseparable from the other parts. It is not possible here to mechanically isolate a part which shall be free from the nervous system as can be done almost completely in the center of the jelly-fish and the apex of the heart. We are dealing with an entire organ which must be considered as an indicator by which comparative results may be obtained. So many un-. known conditions exist in such an organ that it is impossible to say what tissue is acted on primarily, whether the nervous system on the one hand, or the glandular and muscular tissues on the other. There are, however, two indicators in the intestine by which the comparative actions of substances can be studied, namely, the muscular movements, and the secretion of fluid, both of which by various chemical substances may be increased or lessened; or, in other words, they may be stimulated or inhibited. These terms are entirely comparative. The fact that calcium and magnesium act as inhibitors for both the muscular and secretory activities of the intestine does not imply that they have a similar action in other organs or in all animals. It can only be said with certainty that the chemical conditions under which the intestines of the rabbit live are fairly constant, so that the addition of calcium or magnesium in some way constantly inhibits the activity of both muscular and glandular tissues, and the addition of certain purgative salts constantly stimulates them to greater activity.

CHAPTER VI.

The Action of Saline Solutions on Loops of Intestine Removed from the Body.

The fact shown above that local application of saline solutions to the peritoneal surfaces of the intestine could call forth not only muscular movements of the intestine, but also an increased secretion, suggested the possibility of experimenting with loops of intestine entirely removed from the body. Loops thus isolated are necessarily placed under new conditions differing entirely from those under which loops normally connected exist. As mentioned in an early chapter, it was stated by Claude Bernard that section of the spinal cord below the phrenic causes active movements to appear in the intestine; and it was later shown by Pflüger that section of the splanchnic nerves has the same effect, and stimulation of the peripheral cut ends caused the movements to cease. It was also noticed by van Braam-Houckgeest that although loops of the intestine normally connected in the body remained at rest when immersed in isotonic NaCl solution, active movements appear in the loops when the splanchnic nerves are cut. Moreau further showed that section of the mesenteric nerves causes a large increase in the fluid secreted into the intestine.

I have confirmed these results and have found that loops which are quiet when the abdomen is opened remain quiet when placed in m/6 NaCl solution. If, however, loops have become active in any way, through exposure to the air, or through any stimulation, these movements continue when the loops are placed in the salt solution. In any case section of the cervical cord or of the splanchnic nerves, or clamping of the nerves and bloodvessels supplying the loops, causes a very marked increase in the peristaltic activity of the loops. In studying the behavior of isolated loops removed from the body and placed in various solutions it was therefore necessary to consider the effects produced by the removal itself.

In describing these experiments, which were made some time ago,[59] a word may be said as to the methods employed. The rabbits were anaesthetized with morphine as described before; the abdominal cavity was opened and the bloodvessels supplying the loop selected were carefully tied off. Two pairs of ligatures were then placed around the intestine so that the loop was properly isolated. The intestine was then cut between each pair of ligatures, and the mesentery divided between the bloodvessel ligatures and the intestine. In this way the loop could be taken from the body without injuring it, and without causing the animal to lose more than a drop or two of blood. The loop was then emptied by cutting one ligature and allowing the fluid to drain from that end while it was held up by the ligature of the other end. The open end was then religatured, and the whole loop suspended in the solution to be tested. This was arranged so that both ends of the loop were above the surface of the solution, in order that none of the solution could by any possibility enter the lumen of the loop through the ligatured ends. The beakers containing the solutions were kept in a water bath at 39.5° C. The movements of the loops could in this way be directly watched, and the amount of fluid secreted in a unit of time could be easily measured.

If a loop such as has been described above be removed from the intestine of a rabbit and placed in m/8–m/6 NaCl solution at body temperature, active movements at once appear. These are regular and rhythmical, resembling those which set in when the nerves to the intestine

[59] MacCallum, J. B.: University of California Publications, Physiology, Vol. I, 1904, p. 115.

are cut in the uninjured animal. If the loop be allowed to lie at the bottom of the solution, it will twist and writhe about in a peculiar worm-like manner. These movements persist in varying intensity for a considerable time, sometimes as long as an hour, usually for 40–45 minutes. They disappear gradually. No attempt was made to obtain a fluid in which the movements could be maintained for a longer time. These movements are probably merely the continuation of those always caused by sectioning the nerves to the loop. The m/6 or m/8 NaCl solution seems to be fairly favorable for their maintenance. That the loop, however, is not dead when the movements in NaCl cease is shown by the fact that it can be caused to exhibit active movements by transferring it to a solution of NaCl containing a small quantity of BaCl$_2$. It is of course not possible to say that the movements which appear when the loop is placed in pure NaCl solution are entirely due to the cutting of the nerves to the loop. It is possible that the NaCl acts as a direct stimulus and causes the movements to continue.

When a loop is carefully emptied and suspended in a solution of m/8–m/6 NaCl in the way described, it is found that after a considerable time (20–40 minutes) it is still quite empty. If, on the other hand, an m/2 solution of NaCl is used the loop is found to contain after 15 to 20 minutes a small but distinct quantity of clear yellowish fluid resembling the normal intestinal juice. A loop 27 cm. long suspended in m/2 NaCl for 20 minutes contained 0.6 c.c. fluid. A second loop 30 cm. long in the same solution contained 0.8 c.c. fluid. A control loop of the same length in m/8 NaCl remained empty. In m/2 NaCl the movements of the loop are spasmodic and the contractions very strong. The movements do not usually last more than 5 minutes, although the loop may be removed from this solution 15 minutes after the movements have ceased, and may be caused to move again by immersing it in m/8 NaCl containing 1/25 of its volume of m/8 $BaCl_2$. This shows that the loop is not actually killed by the strong NaCl solution.

A loop suspended in m/6 sodium citrate solution showed active peristaltic movements, lasting for 20 to 30 minutes. No fluid, however, collected in this loop. When suspended, however, in m/2 sodium citrate a measurable quantity of fluid was obtained after 20 minutes. A similar result was obtained with Na_2SO_4, active peristalsis, but no secretion being caused in an m/6 solution. In an m/2 solution, however, a considerable quantity of fluid collected in the loop.

A loop 28 cm. long suspended in m/8 NaF exhibited active peristaltic movements which continued for less than 10 minutes. At the end of 20 minutes the loop was found to contain 0.8 c.c. of a clear but slightly blood-stained fluid.

Loops suspended in m/6 NaCl containing m/6 or m/8 $BaCl_2$ in the proportion of 50 to 1 or 70 to 1 showed very strong muscular contractions and a well marked secretion of fluid. The muscular movements were characteristic of barium. Violent local contractions and firm constrictions of the intestine together with strong peristaltic movements took place. The loops always contained a distinct and measurable quantity of fluid after being suspended in this fluid, as may be seen in the table which follows.

Loops placed in m/6 $CaCl_2$ showed no muscular movements whatever, nor did any fluid gather in the lumen. This is in marked contrast to the behavior of the loops in the solutions already described. In equal parts of m/6 NaCl and m/6 $CaCl_2$ no movements or secretion took place.

The results of a number of these experiments may be observed in the following table:—

No.	Salt	Concentration of Solution	Time	Length of loop	Muscular movements and duration	
1	NaCl	m/8	40 min.	30 cm.	Active peristalsis 40 min.	0.0
2	"	"	20 "	23 "	Active peristalsis 40 min.	0.0
3	"	m/2	20 "	30 "	Strong contractions 5 min.	0.8 c.c. clear ye low fluid.
4	"	"	20 "	30 "	Strong contractions 5 min.	0.6 c.c. clear ye low fluid.
5	Sod. Cit.	m/8	20 "		Active peristalsis 20 min.	0.0
		m/2	20 "		Violent contractions 2-3 min.	0.4 c.c. clear ye low fluid.
7	Na$_2$SO$_4$	m/8	20 "		Active peristalsis	0.0
3	"	m/2	20 "		Strong contractions of short duration.	1.5 c.c. clear ye low fluid.
9	Na F	m/8	20 "		Strong contractions 10 min.	
10	{ NaCl BaCl$_2$	m/8-70 c.c. m/8- 1 c.c.	20 "		Active mov'm'ts.	0.6 c.c. clear ye low fluid.
11	"	"	20 "		Active mov'm'ts.	0.8 c.c.
12			20 "		Active mov'm'ts.	1.2 c.c.
13	"	"	20 "		Active mov'm'ts.	1.2 c.c.
14	{ NaCl BaCl$_2$	m/8-50 c.c. m/8- 1 c.c.	1st 20 min. 2nd 20 "		Active mov'm'ts.	1.6 c.c. 0.2 c.c.
15	BaCl$_2$	m/8-50 c.c.	1st 20 min. 2nd 20 min.		Violent contractions.	2.7 c.c. 0.2 c.c.
16	{ NaCl BaCl$_2$	m/8-30 c.c. m/8-30 c.c.	20 min.		Violent contractions.	0.9 c.c.
17	CaCl$_2$	m/8	20 "		None	None
18	"	"	20 "		"	"
19	{ CaCl$_2$ NaCl	m/8-50 c.c. m/8-50 c.c.	20 "		"	
20	{ CaCl$_2$ NaCl	m/2-50 c.c. m/2-50 c.c.	20 "		Slight movements not peristaltic in character.	"
21	{ CaCl$_2$ NaCl	m/1-50 c.c. m/1-50 c.c.	20 "		Slight movements not peristaltic in character.	Slight trace.
22	{ NaCl BaCl$_2$ CaCl$_2$	m/8-30 c.c. m/8- 1 c.c. m/8-30 c.c.	20 "		Irregular contractions, not strong	None.
23	{ NaCl BaCl$_2$ CaCl$_2$	m/8-30 c.c. m/8- 1 c.c. m/8-30 c.c.	20 "		Irregular contractions, not strong	0.2 c.c.

It is interesting to note again here that the secretion into these loops is almost uniformly inhibited by the presence of calcium. When barium is also present in the solution this inhibition is only partial. The action of barium is never entirely counteracted by calcium chloride.

The experiments further show that the saline purgatives act on the intestine not only when it has its normal position and connections with the rest of the body, but also when it is entirely isolated. This eliminates in the first place the possibility of the solutions acting entirely through the central nervous system. It is possible that the salts have some influence on the central nervous system, but from these experiments it seems probable that their main action is either on the glandular and muscular tissues themselves, or on the plexuses of Auerbach and Meissner in the intestinal walls.

As I have already shown, the action of a saline purgative on the intestine consists of two parts, the increase of the peristaltic activity and the increase of the· amount of fluid secreted into the lumen; or, in other words, the action on the muscle and the action on the glandular tissue. In the experiments just described it is clear that these two separate actions exist side by side. For example, m/8 solutions of sodium chloride, citrate, or sulphate cause well marked peristaltic movements or allow these to continue, while no secretion of fluid takes place. Stronger solutions of these salts, on the other hand, such as m/2 produce a distinct secretion. Thus a concentration of a salt which is sufficient to produce muscular activity may not be sufficient to affect the glandular tissues. One is tempted to conclude that in the intestine it requires a stronger stimulus to produce secretory activity than it does to cause muscular movements. It is possible that this is true, but the anatomical relations also must be taken into consideration. The muscle coats lie immediately under the thin peritoneal layer through which the salts are absorbed; and it seems probable that in the experiments described the solutions reached the muscle more easily and rapidly than they could the glandular tissue which is situated on the other side of the muscular and submucous layers. Further, it must be noticed that the movements seen in m/8 NaCl may be merely the continuation of those caused by separation of the loop from the central nervous system.

The amount of fluid which may be secreted by a loop of intestine isolated from the body is limited by the absence of the blood supply. The loop, as shown above, secretes a certain amount of fluid in the first 10 or 20 minutes. If it is then emptied, usually no more fluid appears. The quantity secreted depends on the amount of fluid contained in the intestinal walls at the time of its removal from the body. No fluid passes from the solution in which the loop is suspended into the lumen of the loop; no current is established through the walls from the outside inwards. It seems possible to supply the stimulus for secretion in the solution in which the loop is suspended; but it is not possible in this way to renew the fluid which the glands have secreted into the lumen. This can apparently be done only through the blood vessels.

CHAPTER VII.

The Action on the Intestine of Solutions Containing Two Salts.

As stated above, it was shown by Claude Bernard and by Pflüger that section of the spinal cord below the phrenic nerve, or section of the splanchnic nerves, causes a marked increase in the intestinal movements, and also an increase in the amount of fluid secreted (Moreau). These movements continue in loops isolated and removed from the body and placed in m/6 NaCl, LiCl, Na_2SO_4, sodium citrate, etc., for varying periods of time. They continue far longer in NaCl than in any other solution. Calcium chloride inhibits these movements, as is the case also with magnesium chloride. It was found,[60] however, in making these experiments with isolated loops removed from the body, that with certain mixtures of NaCl or LiCl with $CaCl_2$ or $MgCl_2$, movements began after 20 or 25 minutes of a character differing entirely from the movements seen in pure NaCl. An idea of this phenomenon may be gained from the following description of experiments.

A word may be first said with regard to the methods used in these experiments. In rabbits anaesthetized as usual, the abdomen was opened and a loop 30–40 cm. in length isolated by ligatures. By means of a needle and thread the bloodvessels supplying the loop were carefully tied and the loop rapidly excised. It was then cut into a number of pieces, usually four, which were transferred with

---

[60] MacCallum, J. B.: University of California Publications, Physiology, Vol. II, 1905, p. 47.

as little handling as possible to the beakers containing the solutions to be tested. These beakers were kept in a water bath at 39.5° C. It is desirable in these experiments to use loops which contain no faeces, since unknown substances in the faeces might go into solution and disguise the action of the salt being tested. For this reason the upper part of the small intestine was principally used since in the rabbit it is usually empty or can be readily emptied. In each set of experiments the loops must all come from the same rabbit, for there exist considerable differences in irritability in different animals. On account of these differences it is necessary to have control experiments in the case of each rabbit. Loops also which have been unduly exposed to the air cannot be used. It is of great importance to keep the solutions at a constant body temperature.

(a) *LiCl and CaCl$_2$*. A loop of intestine removed from the body and placed in an m/6 LiCl solution at body temperature usually exhibits only slight movements, which soon cease. This seems to vary somewhat with different rabbits. In some cases the loop shows no movements at all, while in other instances it moves regularly for half a minute and then comes to rest in the solution. These movements are quiet and regular and resemble those described in loops immersed in m/6 NaCl solution. When a loop has ceased to move it does not become active again. In exceptional cases these movements may last 5–10 minutes, but rarely longer. The LiCl solution seems less favorable for the long duration of the movements than the NaCl.

A loop similarly immersed in m/6 CaCl$_2$ solution at body temperature remains in the great majority of cases quite motionless from the first. In some instances slight movements appear immediately after it is placed in the solution, but these soon disappear. After 25–40 minutes it is not uncommon to see the loop slowly straighten out, and at the end of this time the length of the loop is much less than it was at first. This seems to be due to a slow contraction of the longitudinal muscle layer, so slow that no movement can be observed. A difference is seen also in the shape of the loops placed in LiCl and in CaCl$_2$. The former after it comes to rest is practically its original length and is coiled up in a circle; the latter is about half its original length and is almost straight.

A loop similar to the above placed in 50 c.c. m/6 LiCl + 5 c.c. m/6 CaCl$_2$ behaves in a manner entirely different from loops from the same animal placed in either LiCl or CaCl$_2$ alone. On being first immersed in the mixture it exhibits practically no movements. Even in cases where the control loop is active at first the corresponding loop in the mixture of LiCl and CaCl$_2$ shows no movements. It remains perfectly quiet for 10–15 minutes. Then sharp constrictions appear here and there in the loop. These are followed a second or two later by violent contractions which cause the loop to coil upon itself in a most active manner. These contractions somewhat resemble those caused by BaCl$_2$ in the intact intestine. They follow one another rapidly so that the loop is turned and twisted tightly upon itself. This extreme activity persists for 30–45 minutes, sometimes for an hour, while during all this time the control loops in LiCl and in CaCl$_2$ are entirely motionless. These movements are not at all of the same character as those which may appear at the beginning in pure LiCl solution, and could not be considered as these same movements delayed. Such an experiment is outlined in the following table:—

Time. Loops placed in solutions at	50 c.c. m/6 LiCl	50 c.c. m/6 LiCl + 5 c.c. m/6 CaCl$_2$	50 c.c. m/6 CaCl$_2$
10:05	no movements	no movements	no movements
10:10	no movements	no movements	no movements
10:15	no movements	no movements	no movements
10:19	no movements	violent movements begin	no movements
10:25	no movements	very active movements	no movements
10:30	no movements	very active movements	no movements
10:45	no movements	very active movements	no movements
10:50	no movements	movement less active	no movements
11:00	no movements	movement very slight	no movements
11:15	no movements	movement almost stopped	no movements
11:20	no movements	no movements	no movements

By varying the proportions of LiCl and $CaCl_2$ the results may be somewhat changed. The characteristic contractions may be obtained with as small a quantity of $CaCl_2$ as in a mixture of 50 c.c. m/6 LiCl + ½ c.c. m/6 $CaCl_2$. The movements, however, last only 5–10 minutes and are less active than in a mixture of 50 LiCl + 5 $CaCl_2$. This latter mixture seems to be perhaps the most favorable, although almost equally powerful contractions are obtained with mixtures containing as much as 10 c.c. $CaCl_2$ to 50 c.c. LiCl. When more $CaCl_2$ than this is added the movements usually appear later and last a much shorter time. With equal parts of LiCl and $CaCl_2$ they cease in 15 to 20 minutes, while in a mixture of 5 c.c. LiCl + 50 c.c. $CaCl_2$ the movements appear late and last only 4 or 5 minutes. The loops in mixtures with relatively much $CaCl_2$ come to rest in the shape characteristic of loops in pure $CaCl_2$. They become shortened and are found to be straightened out at the end of the experiment. Where relatively much LiCl is present the loops remain almost their original length and are usually coiled. This is shown in the following table :—

Time	50 c.c. LiCl	50 c.c. LiCl + 5 c.c. $CaCl_2$	50 c.c. $CaCl_2$ + 5 c.c. LiCl	50 c.c. $CaCl_2$
11:14	Length of loop 10 cm.	Length of loop 10 cm.	Length of loop 10 cm.	Length of loop 10 cm.
11:14	no movements	no movements	no movements	no movements
11:20	no movements	very active movements	no movements	no movements
11:35	no movements	very active movements	movements begin	no movements
11:40	no movements	very active movements	Movements slow	no movements
11:50	no movements	very active movements	no movements	no movements
12:00	no movements	very active movements	no movements	no movements
12:05	no movements	no movements	no movements	no movements
12:10	Length about 8 cm.	Length about 8 cm.	Length about 4 cm.	Length about 4 cm.

These muscular contractions which appear in mixtures of LiCl and $CaCl_2$, and do not appear in either LiCl or in $CaCl_2$ alone, are not the continuation of movements caused by separating the loop from the central nervous system. These latter movements which are sometimes seen for a short time following the immersion of the loop in pure LiCl solution are inhibited by $CaCl_2$. Further, the movements which come on later in mixtures of LiCl and $CaCl_2$ are of entirely different character, being convulsive and violent and many times more powerful than any movements seen in pure LiCl. If they were the movements seen in pure LiCl, only delayed by the $CaCl_2$, they should be more active in solutions containing the least $CaCl_2$. This is not the case, since in a mixture of 50 c.c. LiCl $+$ ½ c.c. $CaCl_2$ they are by no means so active as in 50 c.c. LiCl $+$ 5 c.c. $CaCl_2$. A further experiment shows this still more clearly. A loop placed in 50 c.c. m/6 LiCl was allowed to come to rest, and was left in the solution for 10 minutes. No movements whatever were to be seen at this time. There were then added 5 c.c. m/6 $CaCl_2$ to the LiCl solution containing the motionless loop. Within one minute the loop became violently active in the characteristic way described above. This activity continued for nearly an hour.

In attempting to explain this phenomenon one is tempted to take Loeb's suggestion as to the action of calcium in Gonionemus, namely, that it counteracts the poisonous effect of the sodium chloride. If the LiCl solution were toxic, however, it is difficult to imagine that the loop could be restored suddenly to activity as described above by the addition of a small quantity of $CaCl_2$, after it had lain in pure LiCl solution for 10 minutes. It is also difficult to consider calcium as a stimulating agent in this case, since, as shown above, in all other instances in the intestine it has the opposite action. Also calcium chloride alone in no concentration causes this phenomenon. The action of

$CaCl_2$ in this instance is suggestive of the action of a catalyser, the addition of which enormously hastens some chemical reaction. It is possible that the muscular activity in this case depends on a chemical reaction which is brought about neither by LiCl nor by $CaCl_2$, but by a combination of these two or perhaps by an intermediate product.

Whatever may be the explanation of these phenomena, the fact remains, and is easy of demonstration, that an effect is produced on isolated loops of intestine by a combination of LiCl and $CaCl_2$ which is entirely different from what can be produced by either LiCl or $CaCl_2$ alone.

(*b*) *NaCl* + *CaCl₂*. The phenomena described above as occurring when isolated loops of intestine are immersed in mixtures of LiCl and $CaCl_2$ can be produced also in mixtures of NaCl and $CaCl_2$. The behavior of loops placed in pure $CaCl_2$ and in pure NaCl has been described. In the former the loop remains motionless; in the latter regular rhythmical movements continue for 40 minutes or more.

When, however, a loop is placed in 50 c.c. m/6 NaCl + 10 c.c. m/6 $CaCl_2$ there are no movements whatever to be seen at first. The loops remains quiet for about 10 minutes. The movements which are seen from the beginning in the control loop in pure NaCl solution have apparently been inhibited by the $CaCl_2$ present in the mixture. After 10 minutes, however, the loop gradually becomes very active, and violent contractions appear which are similar to those described as taking place in mixtures of LiCl and $CaCl_2$. The loop becomes much more active than the control loop in pure NaCl. The onset in the LiCl mixture is more sudden, but otherwise the phenomenon is practically the same. The movements in NaCl + $CaCl_2$ persist for 30 or 40 minutes, sometimes for an hour. When the concentration of the $CaCl_2$ in the mixture is relatively great this effect is not obtained. This is shown in the following table:—

Time	50 c.c. NaCl	50 c.c. NaCl + 5 c.c. CaCl$_2$	50 c.c. NaCl + 10 c.c. CaCl$_2$	50 c.c. NaCl + 20 c.c. CaCl$_2$	50 c.c. NaCl + 40 c.c. CaCl$_2$	50 c.c. CaCl$_2$
10:35	quite active	no movements	no movements	no movements	no movements	no movements
10:40	quite active	no movements	no movements	no movements	no movements	no movements
10:45	quite active	slight movements	slight movements	no movements	no movements	no movements
10:50	less active	slight movements	slight movements	no movements	no movements	no movements
10:55	still active	very active	very active	no movements	no movements	no movements
11:00	still active	extremely active	extremely active	no movements	no movements	no movements
11:15	still active	extremely active	extremely active	no movements	no movements	no movements
11:30	almost stopped	extremely active	extremely active	no movements	no movements	no movements
11:45	no movements	movements quieter	movements quieter	no movements	no movements	no movements
11:50	no movements	no movements	no movements	no movements	no movements	no movements

Thus here also, as in the case of LiCl and CaCl$_2$, there are produced effects in mixtures of NaCl and CaCl$_2$ which cannot be brought about by either salt alone. The presence of CaCl$_2$ seems to inhibit the movements which are first present in a loop placed in NaCl solution. When added in small quantities, *e.g.*, not more than 10 c.c. m/6 CaCl$_2$ to 50 c.c. m/6 NaCl, it produces after an interval of 10–15 minutes very violent movements such as are never seen in pure NaCl solution nor in pure CaCl$_2$. When, however, it is added in greater proportion than this, *e.g.*, 20 or more c.c. CaCl$_2$ to 50 c.c. NaCl, all movements are stopped. The explanation of this is no more clear than the similar occurrence in mixtures of LiCl and CaCl$_2$.

If a loop be placed in a mixture of LiCl and NaCl in equal parts, movements appear such as are seen in pure NaCl, but do not persist for so long a time. In the mixture of these two salts no such result is obtained as has been described in mixtures of LiCl and CaCl$_2$ or of NaCl and CaCl$_2$. Mixtures of CaCl$_2$ and MgCl$_2$ also produce no such movements. In these few salts it seems to be a mixture of chlorides of a monovalent with a bivalent metal which produces the extreme activity of the loop, while mixtures of chlorides of two monovalent metals or of two bivalent metals do not bring this about.

CHAPTER VIII.

The Effect on the Intestine of Intravenous Saline Infusions.

It has been frequently observed that a quantity of fluid enters the intestine during the intravenous injection of normal salt solution. According to Dastre and Loye,[61] the fluid injected into the veins is largely eliminated by the kidneys, although these organs may be assisted in this function by the salivary glands and intestine. These authors have found fluid to be present in the intestine of rabbits as well as in the pleural and peritoneal cavities after the injeetion of large quantities of salt solution. They state that in such an intravenous injection diarrhœa often results which may be so pronounced that a clear fluid emerges from the rectum. Knoll[62] also mentions the production of diarrhœa by the injection of large quantities of NaCl solution.

Magnus[63] in his work on the production of oedema of the skin by intravenous infusions of salt solutions shows in his tables that a certain amount of fluid is eliminated by the intestines after the kidneys have been removed. A rabbit with both kidneys removed was infused with 1,500 c.c. normal salt solution; 200 g. were eliminated by the intestine. In a second rabbit 1,010 c.c. of fluid were injected into the veins and 60 g. were eliminated by the intestine.

[61] Arch. de physiol. norm. et path., 4 e série, 2, 1888, p. 93; 5 e série, 1, 1889, p. 253.
[62] Arch. für exp. Path. u. Pharm., Bd. XXXVI, S. 293, 1895.
[63] Arch. für exp. Path. u. Pharm., Bd. XLII, S. 250, 1899.

In a dog 1,760 c.c. were injected and 160 g. eliminated by the intestine.

I have made a number of experiments[64] in which the amount of fluid passing into the intestine during the intravenous injection of large quantities of NaCl solution was determined not only when the kidneys were removed from the circulation, but also when they were active. As shown by the following experiments, the fluid secreted by the intestine increases rapidly when m/8 or m/6 NaCl solution is injected into the blood. Without such an injection or other stimulus very little intestinal juice can be gathered in a time as short as that occupied by the experiments. In a rabbit's small intestine there is usually found between 5 and 10 c.c. fluid, often much less.

Exp. 1. Rabbit. The bloodvessels to the kidneys were tied off and two cannulæ were put into the intestine, one 35 cm. from the pylorus and the other in the lower part of the ileum. Each loop was isolated by ligatures. The upper one was about 30 cm. long and the lower one 42 cm. The upper loop in the beginning contained 5 c.c. fluid, which were removed. The lower loop was empty. During the first hour 100 c.c. m/8 NaCl were forced into the blood and 5.2 c.c. fluid appeared in the upper loop and nothing in the lower loop. During the second hour 240 c.c. NaCl solution were injected and 5.4 c.c. fluid appeared in the upper loop and 13.6 c.c. in the lower loop. During the third hour 160 c.c. NaCl solution were introduced; 6.6 c.c. fluid appeared in the upper loop and 15.5 c.c. in the lower. The infusion was then stopped and 26 c.c. were found in the part of the small intestine not included in the loops. The total amount thus secreted by the intestine in three hours was 72.3 c.c. This is 14.46% of the quantity injected.

Exp. 2. In another rabbit with kidneys removed, 470 c.c. NaCl solution were injected during three hours, and 78

<hr />

[64] MacCallum, J. B.: University of California Publications, Physiology, Vol. I, 1904, p. 125.

c.c. fluid obtained from the intestine, which is about 16.6% of the quantity injected.

Exp. 3. In a rabbit in which the kidneys were left intact, 547 c.c. m/6 NaCl solution were injected into the blood. 49.5 c.c. were secreted in 3 hours and 30 minutes by the intestine. This is about 9% of the total quantity of fluid. The quantity of fluid secreted into the loop in the first half hour was 1.8 c.c.; in the third half hour, 2.9 c.c.; in the fifth half hour, 6.6 c.c.

Exp. 4. In a second rabbit in which the kidneys were untouched, the quantity of m/8 NaCl solution introduced was 390 c.c.; about 40 c.c. of fluid were obtained during three hours from the intestine. This is 10.25% of the amount injected. In the first hour 5 c.c. were secreted into the loop; in the second hour 7 c.c.; and in the third hour 11.1 c.c. In the rest of the small intestine 17 c.c. were found.

It is clear from these experiments that a considerable proportion of the fluid injected in this way is eliminated by the intestine. The quantity is somewhat greater if the kidneys are extirpated. There is, however, a limit to the amount that can be excreted by the intestine, and never, as in the case of the kidney, does the amount excreted approximate the amount injected. The action of such infusions on the intestine is nevertheless quite similar to that on the kidneys, and in many other ways the intestine may be regarded as an excretory organ which can to some extent take on the functions of the kidney. The intestinal juice contains many substances contained by the urine. Among the more conspicuous of these is urea, which was shown by Claude Bernard[65] to be excreted into the intestine as well as the stomach. He found that it is readily broken up in the intestinal juice, so that in many cases only salts of ammonia remain.

---

[65] Leçons sur les propriétés physiologiques et les altérations pathologiques des liquides de l'organisme, II Tome, Paris, 1859. Deuxième Leçon.

Pregl[66] demonstrated the presence of urea in the intestinal juice of the sheep. He found its concentration there to be 0.248%. In the intestinal juice of rabbits I[67] have found that small quantities of urea exist both before and after extirpation of the kidneys. It is present not only in the normal intestinal juice, but also in the fluid obtained from the intestine after the infusion of large quantities of m/6 NaCl. Weintrand[68] has demonstrated uric acid in the intestinal juice.

Secretion of sugar into the intestine. Another instance of the way in which the intestine can to some extent take up the function of the kidney is shown by the secretion of sugar by the gut following the injection of large quantities of normal salt solution. It was shown by Bock and Hoffmann[69] that the injection of 1% NaCl solution into the circulation of a rabbit caused transient glycosuria. Large quantities of the solution were injected at the rate of 25–30 c.c. each 5 minutes, and the glycosuria appeared in from 20 minutes to 1 hour and 30 minutes after the beginning of the infusion. After a number of hours (6–7) the glycosuria diminished in their experiments and finally disappeared, although the infusion of salt and the flow of urine continued. They found that the entire quantity of sugar eliminated was in one case 1.632 g., and in another case 2.04 g. The percentage of sugar in the urine reached 0.136 and 0.219 respectively in the two experiments. These facts were confirmed by Külz,[70] who found also that section of the splanchnics prevented the glycosuria. The experiments lately published by M. H. Fischer[71] show that the glycosuria is caused not only by NaCl, but by certain of the salts

[66] Archiv für die gesammte Physiologie, Bd. 61, 1895, p. 378.
[67] *Loc. cit.*
[68] Chemische Centralblatt, Leipzig, Bd. II, 1895, S. 310.
[69] BOCK and HOFFMANN: Arch. für Anat., Physiol. und wissenschaftl. Med. (Reichert und DuBois-Reymond), p. 550, 1871.
[70] KÜLZ: C. Eckhard's Beiträge, Bd. 6, S. 117, 1872. (Quoted by Pflüger, Arch. für die gesammte Physiologie, Bd. 96, 1903, S. 313.)
[71] M. H. FISCHER: University of California Publications, Physiology, Vol. I, pp. 77 and 87, 1904.

which were shown by Loeb[72] to produce muscular twitch-ings. He further showed that calcium has the power of suppressing the glycosuria.

This secretion of sugar by the kidneys following intra-venous infusions, together with the facts shown above that fluid is eliminated to some extent by the intestine in the absence of the kidneys, led me to inquire whether the in-testine also secretes sugar when the kidneys have been ex-tirpated and a large amount of NaCl solution is injected. A number of experiments were made to determine this. I have found[73] in brief that with the infusion of large quan-tities of m/6 NaCl solution into the circulation sugar is abundantly secreted into the intestine. This takes place not only when the kidneys are removed, but also when they are intact, and are also eliminating sugar. This may be seen in the following tables:—

Rabbit—Blood vessels of kidney ligatured; cannula in upper part of small intestine, with loop 35 cm. tied off. Loop emptied; contents 5 c.c., which contained no sugar.

Time	NaCl m/6 injected	Intestinal juice	Sugar examination of intestinal juice
10:00	Infusion begun	Loop emptied, 5 c.c.	No sugar
10:30	20 c.c.	3 c.c.	No sugar
11:00	40 c.c.	3 c.c.	No sugar
11:30	20 c.c.	4 c.c.	No sugar
12:00	120 c.c.	6 c.c.	Trace of sugar
12:30	200 c.c.	12 c.c.	Sugar abundant
1:00	— c.c.	28 c.c.	Sugar abundant
	400 c.c.		

Here the sugar appeared in the intestinal juice after about 200 c.c. NaCl solution had been injected. The injec-tion was made in each case into the vein of the ear by means

[72] LOEB, J: Festschrift für Fick, 1899; Pflüger's Archiv, 1902, XCI, p. 248.
[73] MACCALLUM, J. B.: University of California Publications, Phys-iology, Vol. I, 1904, p. 125.

of a pressure bottle connected with the water tap. The pressure bottle was in turn connected with a bottle holding the solution, which was thus forced out at a constant rate through a long rubber tube immersed in water at 40° C. A hypodermic needle was fastened in the end of this tube and inserted into the marginal vein of the rabbit's ear. In this way the quantity of fluid injected could be accurately measured and controlled. The salt solution after passing through the long tube reached the ear at approximately body temperature. It is of the greatest importance to protect the intestinal loops in every way possible from loss of heat or from drying.

In the above experiment the *intestinal glycosuria*, if such a term may be applied to this phenomenon, appears under circumstances which are exactly the same as those necessary for the production of sugar in the urine by saline infusions. A further example of this is shown in the following experiment:—

Rabbit—Blood vessels of both kidneys ligatured. Intestinal loop including duodenum 32 cm. long. In the loop were found 3 c.c. fluid which contained no sugar.

Time	NaCl m/6 injected	Intestinal juice	Sugar examination of intestinal juice
9:45	Infusion begun	Loop emptied, 3 c.c.	No sugar
10:15	10 c.c.	3 c.c.	No sugar
10:45	70 c.c.	3 c.c.	No sugar
11:15	75 c.c.	3.2 c.c.	No sugar
11:45	85 c.c.	5 c.c.	Sugar abundant } 0.202% 0.222%
12:15	80 c.c.	9.5 c.c.	Sugar abundant 0.25%
12:45	150 c.c.	21 c.c.	Sugar abundant
	470 c.c.		

Here the sugar appeared after the infusion of about 240 c.c. NaCl solution. The experiment was not carried on to see how long the sugar would continue to be present in the intestinal juice. The animal was killed, and it was found that the remaining loops of the small intestine held 32 c.c. of fluid which contained sugar. The stomach contents included about 40 c.c. fluid which also contained sugar. Of the 470 c.c. of fluid injected, 78.7 c.c. were eliminated by the small intestine and 40 by the stomach. The alimentary canal, then, exclusive of the large intestine, eliminated about 118 c.c. of the fluid introduced, which is approximately 25%.

Quantitative estimations of the sugar in the intestinal juice in this case were made. The amount varied between 0.2 and 0.3%. I have not attempted to ascertain the total quantity of sugar which may be obtained from the intestinal juice by continued infusion of salt solution. In the case of the urine, Bock and Hoffmann made such determinations and found that the kidney eliminated in one case 1.632 g. and in another case 2.04 g. sugar. M· H. Fischer found that the concentration of sugar in the urine of a rabbit rarely exceeds 0.25% after infusion of m/6 NaCl.

Thus the intestine eliminates sugar in a way that entirely resembles its elimination by the kidneys. The sugar appears in the blood after the infusion of a certain amount of the salt solution and is excreted by the kidney. If the kidneys are removed, it is excreted by the intestine. But even when the kidneys are intact there is a certain amount of sugar excreted by the intestine, just as a part of the fluid injected is eliminated by the intestine when the kidneys are still active. As shown in the following experiment, the sugar appears both in the intestinal juice and in the urine. The quantity of sugar, however, is greater in the urine than in the intestinal juice. In the urine it was found to be about 0.2%, in the intestinal juice considerably less. The quantity of urine also is greater than the quantity of intestinal juice. Therefore the greater proportion of the sugar is excreted by the kidneys.

Rabbit—Cannula placed in bladder. Kidneys intact. Cannula in loop of upper part of small intestine 35 cm. long. Loop contained 4.2 c.c. fluid; no sugar.

Time.	$NaCl\frac{m}{6}$ injected.	Intestinal juice.		Urine.	
		Quantity.	Sugar examination.	Quantity.	Sugar examination.
9:45	Infusion begun.	Loop emp'd, 4.2 c.c.	No sugar.	Bladder emptied, 5 c.c.	No sugar.
10:15	5 c.c.	1.8 c.c.	" "	0.0	
10:45	50 "	2.2 "		0.0	
11:15	80 "	2.9 "		4.0 c.c.	No sugar.
11:45	92 "	3.8 "	" "	15.0	Sugar present.
12:15	120 "	6.6 "	Sugar present.	38.0	Much sugar.
12:45	150 "	7.8 "	" "	40.0	" "
	497 "				

It is interesting to note in connection with these experiments the secretion of sugar into the stomach which followed the intravenous infusion of NaCl solution. Ordinarily in the normal rabbit only a very small quantity of fluid can be obtained from the stomach. This was not found in my experiments to contain sugar. In one case after the infusion of 470 c.c. NaCl solution the stomach contained about 40 c.c. of fluid. In a second instance 32.8 c.c. of fluid were secreted by the stomach during 2 hours and 30 minutes, during which time 390 c.c. NaCl solution were injected. In both these experiments sugar, which was not present in the beginning, appeared in considerable quantities after the infusion had continued for a little time. Thus the stomach excretes sugar under circumstances similar to those under which it is excreted by the intestine. Claude Bernard[74] describes the presence of sugar in the gastric contents of diabetic patients. He quotes McGregor as having made the observation by causing patients to vomit. On examination of the gastric contents sugar was demonstrated. It seems possible that in this case the food might have contained a reducing substance.

[74] Leçons sur les propriétés physiologiques des liquides de l'organisme, T. II, 1859, p. 74.

Thus a study of the effect of saline infusions on the intestine leads us to the idea of the alimentary canal as in some sense a subsidiary excretory organ. In addition to its other better known functions, the intestine can to some extent take on some of the functions of the kidney. As shown above, it not only tends to eliminate an excess of fluid forced into the circulation, but also excretes urea and uric acid. Further, under circumstances which cause glycosuria, sugar is also excreted by the intestine.

CHAPTER IX.

Mode of Action of the Saline Cathartics.

Since the discovery of sodium sulphate by Glauber in the middle of the seventeenth century, and the preparation of the double tartrate of sodium and potassium at Rochelle some fifteen years later, the saline cathartics have been in constant use among physicians. Attempts have been made also from the first to explain in some way their mode of action; but it was not until the discovery of the osmotic property of salts that any explanation which seemed satisfactory was made. Poiseuille[75] and Liebig[76] both advanced the theory that the purgative action of salts was due to their power of attracting water into the lumen of the intestine, *i.e.*, to their power of endosmosis. This seemed at first sight to be very satisfactory and to account well for the increased amount of fluid in the faeces following the administration of a saline cathartic. The theory did not, however, take into consideration other substances whose osmotic power is as great as that of the purgative salts, but which have no purgative action whatever. It was later, however, supported by Rabuteau[77] in an experiment in which he claimed to have found that the intravenous injection of a large quantity of sodium sulphate produced constipation, while the same salt given by mouth causes purgation. This he ascribed to the flow of fluid towards the salt in each case due to its osmotic

[75] Recherch. expériment. sur les mouvements des liquides dans les tubes de petits diamètres, Paris, 1828. Quoted from Hay.
[76] Über die Saftbewegung, 1848.
[77] L'Union médicale, 1871, 50, 51. Gaz méd. de Paris, 1879.

pressure. This experiment lacks confirmation, and indeed it has been shown above that sodium sulphate and other saline cathartics produce increased peristalsis and in some cases increase of fluid in the intestine when introduced intravenously or applied on the serous surfaces of the intestine. And these evidences of a purgative action appear much more rapidly and with smaller doses than when the salt is placed in the lumen of the intestine. Claude Bernard[78] states in his criticism of this theory that the intravenous injection of sodium sulphate causes purgation, and further draws attention to the fact that on this theory of the endosmotic action of cathartics, sugar, which has a high osmotic power, should be among the more powerful purgatives. It was further shown by other investigators that of several purgative salts, the most powerful was not the one with the highest osmotic power.

Headland,[79] believing that all medicines must first pass into the circulation before they act, claimed that the saline purgatives are absorbed from the intestine and are again excreted lower down in the intestine, and in being excreted they stimulate the glands to secrete.

A little later than this it was shown by Moreau[80] and others that solutions of purgative salts placed in loops of intestine which had been tied off caused an increased secretion of fluid into the intestine. Brieger[81] further confirmed this with better methods and showed that the fluid was a real secretion, and not an inflammatory exudate, or a transudation.

Thiry in a series of experiments was unable to produce increased secretion of fluid from a Thiry-Vella fistula by the introduction of sulphate of magnesia. He therefore concludes that the action of saline cathartics is due solely

[78] Substances toxiques et médicamenteuses, 1857.
[79] Action of Medicines, 1867.
[80] Archiv. général d. médicine, VI Série f. XVI, 1870. Centralbl. f. d. medicin. Wiss., 1868, p. 209.
[81] Arch. f. exp. Path. u. Pharm., Bd. VIII, 1878, S. 355.

to an increase in peristaltic activity. Radziejewski[82] held a similar theory and made many experiments in an attempt to prove that an increase in peristaltic activity was the main result of the administration of a saline purgative. In connection with this it may be noted that van Braam-Houckgeest[83] concluded from his experiments that saline purgatives do not increase the peristaltic activity of the intestine. It is difficult to imagine how these results could be obtained.

Hay[84] quotes Aubert, Buchheim, and Wagner as holding the theory that in addition to causing an increased peristalsis, the salt is slowly absorbed, and tends to prevent the absorption of fluid from the intestine. This theory was held also by Schmiedeberg,[85] who claimed that the purgative salts were absorbed with difficulty and reached the lower parts of the intestine unchanged. In the large intestine the salts, according to this hypothesis, prevent the faeces from becoming compact by inhibiting the absorption of water from the lumen. This explanation of the action of cathartic salts has been widely accepted and has been supported by Wallace and Cushny,[86] who claim in addition that the salts of acids which form insoluble compounds with calcium are especially active in inhibiting the absorption of fluids from the intestine.

Loeb in studying the action of salts in the production of muscular twitchings in voluntary muscles, and of hypersensitiveness of the skin and nervous elements, recognized the fact that the salts which had these actions included those commonly known as saline purgatives. He says in this connection: "I will not deny the effect of these salts upon the phenomena of absorption of water from the intestine, but it is obvious from our experiments that the same salts must increase the irritability of the nerves and muscles of the

---

[82] Reichert's u. DuBois-Reymond's Archiv, 1870, S. 37.
[83] Pflüger's Archiv, 1872, S. 266.
[84] Loc. cit.
[85] Arzneimittellehre, Leipzig, 1883.
[86] Amer. Journ. Physiol., 1898, Vol. I, p. 411.

intestine, and that this must facilitate the production of peristaltic motions, possibly through the mechanical or contact stimuli of the faeces upon the nerve endings or the muscular wall of the intestine.''[87]

My own experiments which I have described above support this suggestion of Loeb's. In the first place it was found that the subcutaneous or intravenous injection of one of these salts, especially sodium citrate, caused muscular twitchings in the living rabbit. This had already been done by Loeb in the frog. In both cases the injection of calcium chloride inhibits the twitchings. As shown above, there are produced in a rabbit by such an injection of a purgative salt not only muscular twitchings, but also increased peristaltic movements, and an increased flow of fluid into the intestine. The subsequent injection of calcium chloride was shown to inhibit both the increased secretion and the increased movements of the intestine. There thus seems to be a very distinct analogy between the action of these salts in producing twitchings in voluntary muscles and the production of their purgative effect; and a similar analogy between the suppression of the former and the suppression of the latter by calcium chloride. One is tempted to suppose that these purgative salts act by removing calcium from the tissues, as suggested by Loeb, in the production of muscular twitchings, since they are all calcium precipitants. There is, however, no direct proof of this, and other saline purgatives such as $BaCl_2$ and Hg_2Cl_2 certainly have an action which is independent of calcium.

There thus seems to be produced by saline purgatives a condition of increased irritability in the intestine analogous to the increased irritability produced in the voluntary muscles. As a result of this the two main activities of the intestine are increased, namely, the peristaltic activity and the secretory activity. The action of the saline purgative,

---

[87] LOEB: Decennial Publications, University of Chicago, Vol. X, 1902, p. 10.

then, as far as we know, consists of two main parts. The peristaltic movements are greatly increased in rapidity and force, and the faeces are carried rapidly from the upper to the lower parts of the intestine. They are thus passed through the large intestine in so short a time that the fluid they already contain has not time in which to be reabsorbed, a process which apparently takes place normally in the large intestine. At the same time there is a much larger quantity of fluid secreted into the lumen of the intestine than takes place in the normal animal. The faeces which are thus forced rapidly through the gut by the increased peristaltic movements are more fluid than normal. This together with the rapid passage of the faeces accounts for their fluid character when a saline purgative is given.

Whether or not the saline purgatives also inhibit the absorption of fluid from the intestine cannot be stated with certainty. The experiments of Wallace and Cushny leave out of account the increased secretion of fluid into the intestine caused by the purgative, a process which undoubtedly takes place. Thus in comparing the amount of NaCl, and the amount of a saline purgative absorbed in a given time from separate loops under the same conditions, it is not surprising that the amount of NaCl solution found in the loop after the experiment is less than the amount of purgative solution left. If the quantities of the two salts were equal in the beginning and an equal amount were absorbed, there would still be more fluid left in the loop containing the purgative on account of the secretion of fluid into the loop which was caused by the purgative, and not by the NaCl.

With regard to the mode in which the salt must be administered it is quite clear that it is not necessary to place it in the stomach or the lumen of the intestine. As shown above, the action is more rapid and more powerful when the solution is injected into the blood, or applied locally to the peritoneal surface of the intestine. Nor is the action due to its being secreted again into the lumen of the intestine, because the action is almost immediate when the solution is poured on the outside of the loops, and only takes place after several minutes when placed in the lumen. If injected into the blood the action is slower than when the solution is applied to the serous surfaces of the intestine. In the former case every opportunity would be afforded for its rapid excretion into the intestine if that were a factor. It is evident that the solution must be absorbed into the blood and bathe the tissues just as a solution surrounds a muscle which is immersed in it.

As to the tissues in the intestine which are primarily affected, it is impossible to make a definite statement. The muscle and glands cannot be at all separated from the complex nervous mechanism of the intestine, and it is necessary to take the whole as an organ made up of many tissues and affected in definite ways by certain solutions.

It is interesting in this connection to again note the effect of these salts on the secretion of urine. It is well known that practically all of them are diuretics, when introduced with a considerable amount of fluid. And even when the flow of urine has been greatly increased by the injection of $m/6$ NaCl solution, it can be still further augmented by the addition of, e.g., sodium citrate to the injection fluid. These salts constitute the well known class of saline diureties. All salts do not, however, belong to this class, as is often stated. Calcium chloride, magnesium chloride, and to some extent strontium chloride exert exactly the opposite effect, inhibiting the action of the diuretics and diminishing the flow of urine. These salts might be termed antidiuretics. There is thus an entire analogy between the action of the saline diuretics on the kidney and that of the saline purgatives on the intestine, and also the action of calcium and magnesium is the same in both cases. And the analogy can be traced farther back to the production and inhibition of muscular twitchings in voluntary muscles, which was demonstrated by Loeb.

The actual mechanism of the secretion of fluid into the intestine is difficult to determine. It seems improbable that a change in blood pressure plays any very important rôle, if indeed it has an influence at all. There is much evidence to show that many glands consisting of cells resembling those of the intestine roughly, secrete their characteristic fluids quite independently of blood pressure. In *Sida crystallina,* a small fresh-water crustacean, it was found[88] that if a small quantity of one of the saline purgatives or of $BaCl_2$ or pilocarpine be added to the water in which these crustaceans are lying, there is not only a rapid increase of intestinal movement and a rapid evacuation of faeces, but there is also an increased secretion of fluid into the intestine, so that the whole lumen becomes filled with a pale greenish fluid. It was pointed out further that in this organism there is no closed blood vascular system, the blood simply running in wide channels in more or less definite directions. There can therefore exist nothing here comparable with the blood pressure of higher animals, and yet secretion normally takes place without changes in blood pressure. Further, it can be greatly increased by chemicals without an increase in blood pressure being possible. A similar secretion without blood pressure as a causative factor is seen in the skin of the common slug (Ariolimax). Here the secretion of the skin may be markedly increased by the injection or local application of a solution of any of the saline purgatives. This takes place equally well when the heart of the animal is removed, and also in an isolated portion of the animal, or in a piece of the skin cut off with the scissors. In these latter cases there can be no possibility of blood pressure taking a part in the secretion.

It has been further shown[89] that loops of intestine entirely removed from the body may be caused to secrete a

[88] MacCALLUM, J. B.: University of California Publications, Physiology, Vol. II, 1905, p. 65.
[89] MacCALLUM, J. B.: University of California Publications, Physiology, Vol. I, 1904, p. 115.

measurable quantity of fluid by immersing them in certain purgative solutions, especially those containing $BaCl_2$. Other solutions such as pure m/6 NaCl do not cause this secretion, although active peristaltic movements go on in NaCl. In this case the secretion must be entirely independent of the blood pressure. Pilocarpine also in the salivary gland causes an enormous increase in the secretion, without raising the blood pressure in the carotid.

It is certain from these facts that in many glands secretion is quite independent of any change in blood pressure; and it seems probable that such changes must play a very subordinate part in the secretion of fluid from the intestine.

On the other hand, it is to be noted that in many instances muscular and secretory activities are controlled by the same conditions. There seems to be a common factor in the production of the two functions. Saline purgatives produce not only muscular activity, but also increased secretion; and calcium and magnesium are capable of inhibiting both. Atropin also quiets the movements of the intestine, and at the same time is conspicuous in suppressing the secretion. Section of the splanchnic nerves causes not only increased muscular movements, but an increased secretion of fluid in the intestine. These instances could be greatly increased in number. From them it seems that something exists in common in muscular movements and in glandular activity. What first suggests itself is that the gland cells themselves are made to contract rhythmically by the various conditions which cause rhythmical contractions in muscle. That the stimulus for this must be greater in the case of secretion is shown by the fact that in the intestine peristaltic movements may be maintained in a solution (m/6 NaCl) in which no secretion takes place. It seems not at all improbable that one factor in the production of secretory activity is dependent on a property of the gland cell closely related to muscular contractility.

A further factor is suggested by the action of certain diuretics. In the kidney the changes in the quantity of blood flowing through the organ and to some extent changes in blood pressure influence the flow of urine. The diuresis produced by such substances, however, as saponin, digitalin, potassium chlorate, etc., probably depends on an increase in permeability of the capsule of Bowman. As shown[90] recently, these substances produce haemolysis, and are also strong diuretics. Calcium chloride, which inhibits the flow of urine produced by them, inhibits also the haemolysis. Haemoglobinuria, which readily appears with small doses of saponin or digitalin, is inhibited by simultaneously injecting calcium chloride. There thus seems to be something in common between haemolysis and diuresis; and what suggests itself as most probable is that the permeability of the red blood corpuscle, as well as that of the kidney cell is increased, so that on the one hand haemoglobin escapes into the blood (is secreted into the blood), and the amount of urine on the other hand passing through the kidney cell is increased. Calcium, according to the same idea, would decrease the permeability in both cases.

In secretion we have therefore among other things two factors which probably play a rôle, namely, a property of the gland cell resembling that of muscular contractility and controlled in many cases by the same conditions, and a change in permeability of the cells which are secreting. In the kidney there is a third factor dependent on the flow of blood through the organ. A continuous supply of blood is of course necessary in all glands for a continued secretion.

[90] MacCallum, J. B.: University of California Publications, Physiology, Vol. II, 1905, p. 93.

CHAPTER X.

Possible Therapeutic Value of These Experiments.

It at once suggests itself to the physician that some clinical use might be made of the facts outlined above. If such striking results can be obtained in a rabbit it is possible that some modifications of the use of these saline purgatives might be made in the human being.

If in the first place it is found that subcutaneous or intravenous injections of saline purgatives are effective in man, there arise in both medical and surgical practice occasions in which these methods of administration would be of the greatest advantage. It is to be remembered in this connection that the administration by these methods of $MgSO_4$ is especially dangerous. This salt when rapidly absorbed seems to be very poisonous. Rabbits frequently die in a few minutes after an intravenous injection of a quantity relatively small as compared with the amount of Na_2SO_4 which can be given in this way. Barium chloride is extremely active as a subcutaneous purgative, but should be used with the greatest caution and in very minute quantities on account of its very poisonous character. I can give no idea of the dose that might be given to a human being without danger. A rabbit usually does not recover from a subcutaneous injection of 3 c.c. m/8 BaCl solution.

The fact that saline purgative solutions applied to the peritoneal surfaces of the intestine act very rapidly may suggest some use in abdominal surgery for this method. If it were desirable to have evacuation of the bowel rapidly follow an abdominal operation this procedure might be resorted to. An isotonic solution (m/6) of sodium sulphate or sodium citrate would be most favorable for this purpose.

The possible uses to which our knowledge of the action of calcium may be put has aroused some discussion. The fact that it suppresses muscular and nervous irritability (Loeb), and as shown in the experiments above, inhibits the muscular and glandular activity of the intestine, as well as the secretory activity of the kidney, makes it seem probable that some practical use may be made of it in certain conditions in the human being. The most important of these conditions is perhaps the persistent diarrhœa which sometimes accompanies disorders of an hysterical or neurasthenic sort. There have already come under my notice several cases of diarrhœa of nervous origin which were quite uncontrolled by morphine preparations. These cases were apparently entirely relieved by calcium chloride given for only a few days. (grs XX t.i.d.) Whether a large number of similar patients will show the same results remains to be seen. The treatment is evidently to be applied to only a small class of patients, roughly those cases of persistent diarrhœa of apparently nervous origin, which cannot be influenced by opiates.

When rectal infusions of NaCl are not retained it is possible by adding $CaCl_2$ to the solution to stop the movements of the rectum which cause their expulsion. Enemata of NaCl containing $CaCl_2$ are retained much better than those of pure NaCl.

The marked action of calcium on the kidney suggests that certain conditions might arise where it could be made use of. In nervous polyuria it can be given with benefit; and although we know practically nothing as to the etiology of diabetes insipidus, it is possible that calcium might be employed with advantage to stop the abnormal flow of urine.

With regard to general conditions such as the muscular

and nervous irritability accompanying hysterical and neuraesthenic disturbances little can be said as to the possible value of calcium. Loeb drew attention to the possibilities of its being of use in these diseases, but there is not sufficient evidence to make any statement concerning it. The extreme irritability which is present in some types of insanity might also be tested in this respect.

Calcium might also be of benefit in asthma where the two distressing symptoms are spasmodic contractions of the bronchioles and a hypersecretion from the mucous membrane of the larger and smaller bronchi. Judging by analogy from the experiments described above, calcium should not only relieve the muscular contractions but also inhibit the secretion.

These suggestions are made simply in the hope of stimulating clinical research in this direction.

Wright has recently stated that calcium relieves urticaria, a circumstance which he refers to the influence of calcium on the coagulability of the blood, which he says is diminished in this condition. It seems more probable from the above experiments that the calcium inhibits the secretion or passage of fluid from the lymph vessels to form the vesicles.

CHAPTER XI.

The Action of Purgatives of Vegetable Origin.

This group of purgatives, as far as its general properties are concerned, is so well described in many text-books that it is unnecessary here to go into the details of their preparation and the commoner characteristics of each. Certain points which have come up in connection with my own experiments, however, may be briefly described here.

Cascara Sagrada is prepared in many ways, but the most favorable preparation for experiment is the dried extract. This is the dark yellow powder familiar in commerce. It is found that in shaking this powder in distilled water it is almost entirely insoluble. The result is a dirty yellow mixture, the filtrate from which gives an acid reaction. This suggested neutralizing the mixture or making it alkaline. A small amount of sodium bicarbonate was added, and the powder immediately went into solution, producing a clear dark brown fluid.[92] A similar result was obtained by adding sodium hydrate. It was found that $\frac{1}{2}$ g. of the dried extract could be dissolved in 25 c.c. m/24 $NaHCO_3$. This solution in $NaHCO_3$ is practically neutral. If a few drops of dilute H_2SO_4 be added a yellow precipitate at once appears giving a mixture or suspension similar to that originally obtained by adding the powder to distilled water. The addition of $NaHCO_3$ will again produce the characteristic dark brown solution. The extract is much more readily soluble in a stronger solution of $NaHCO_3$.

[92] MacCallum, J. B.: University of California Publications, Physiology, Vol. I, p. 163.

The dried extract is thus soluble only in a neutral or alkaline fluid. It is insoluble in distilled water on account of the free acid which is present in the powder.

Cascara extract is readily soluble in the intestinal juice of·a rabbit, a characteristic dark brown clear solution being obtained. On the other hand, it is insoluble in the gastric juice, and an alkaline solution added to the gastric juice is at once precipitated.

It was found that the intravenous injection of 1 c.c. of a 2% solution of cascara extract in $m/25$ $NaHCO_3$ produces within a minute very strong peristaltic movements in the intestine. A similar injection of the same amount of $m/25$ $NaHCO_3$ alone produces no such result, though stronger solutions of $NaHCO_3$ cause a slight increase in intestinal movements. It is therefore the cascara in solution which produces these strong contractions.

A somewhat larger quantity of the cascara solution injected subcutaneously produces increased peristaltic activity after an interval of several minutes.

If the cascara solution be applied directly to the serous surfaces of the intestine, very strong contractions and peristaltic movements result in 2 or 3 minutes. A solution of $m/25$ $NaHCO_3$ alone produces very slight movements when applied in this way. These can, however, be readily distinguished from those produced by cascara. The latter are much more powerful, are slower in developing, and can be only partially inhibited by $m/6$ $CaCl_2$. The movements following the application of pure $NaHCO_3$ solution, however, are weak, they appear almost immediately, and can be entirely suppressed by the application of $m/6$ $CaCl_2$ solution.

When the cascara solution is placed in the stomach no movements appear in the intestine even after 15–30 minutes. The acid of the gastric juice has evidently precipitated the cascara, which cannot act until it is passed on into the intestine where it may be dissolved in the alkaline juice of the intestine. If instead of placing the solution in the stomach it is injected directly into the small intestine, increased peristaltic movements begin within 5 minutes. Here it evidently remains in solution and is absorbed. It is for this reason that in human beings cascara taken by mouth acts only after several hours. It is precipitated in the stomach and must reach the intestine before it is dissolved and absorbed.

In addition to the increased peristaltic activity caused by the cascara, there seems to be also an increase in the secretion of fluid into the lumen. One or two hours after the injection 20–30 c.c. fluid could be collected from the small intestine. Without the purgative it is rarely possible to obtain more than 5 to 10 c.c.

It was found that calcium chloride has only a very transient effect in inhibiting the increased movements produced by cascara. For 2 or 3 minutes following the injection of $CaCl_2$ the movements were usually quieted, but they rapidly began again and continued as vigorously as before.

The behavior of rhubarb is in every way similar to that of cascara. It is less readily soluble, but the solution acts in a way quite like that described for cascara.

It is further well known that aloin injected subcutaneously causes increased peristalsis. A study has recently been made of certain constituents of the derivatives of the aloes group of purgatives. Esselmont,[93] following the work of Tschirch,[94] experimented with a number of substances obtained from these purgatives. Aloëemodin is present not only in aloes, but also in Cascara sagrada and senna leaves. A small amount of this substance acts as a purgative. Alochrysin, aloingrin, barbaloin, all act as purgatives. Chrysophanic acid, which is found in aloes, rhubarb, and senna is a mild purgative. It is of interest to note that each of these substances is either a di- or tri-oxymethylanthrachinon. They owe their purgative action, according to

---

[93] Archiv f. exp. Path. u. Pharm., Bd. 43, 1900, S. 274.

[94] Schweiz. Wochenschrift für Chemie und Pharmacie, 1898, No. 23.

Tschirch, to their containing the oxymethylanthrachinon group.

Some experiments[95] which I recently made on a jelly-fish (Polyorchis) with some of the vegetable purgatives are of interest. They were suggested by the experiments of Loeb[96] on the effect of various salts on the isolated center of the animal and of a related form (Gonionemus). When separated from the margins the bell-like centers of these jellyfish do not beat in pure sea-water. In case of Gonionemus it was found that the addition of one of a number of salts (calcium precipitants) caused the center to beat. This group of salts includes the so-called saline purgatives.

The methods used in the experiments with vegetable purgatives were practically the same as those used by Loeb. The animal was bisected just above the ring of sense organs in order to entirely remove the margin containing the main nervous system. The center was then placed in mixtures of sea-water and solutions of the purgatives. The center never beats in pure sea-water, but was found to beat vigorously in sea-water to which a small quantity of a solution of cascara, rhubarb, aloin, podophyllin, or colocynth had been added. It was necessary to dissolve the cascara and rhubarb extracts in $m/24$ $NaHCO_3$, since they are not soluble in pure water. The centers do not beat in sea-water to which pure $m/24$ $NaHCO_3$ has been added in quantities equivalent to those added with the purgative solution.

A solution of $\frac{1}{4}$ g. cascara extract was made in 50 c.c. $m/24$ $NaHCO_3$. It was found that a mixture of 25 c.c. sea-water $+$ 2 c.c. of this cascara solution was the most favorable for producing rhythmical contractions in the isolated center of Polyorchis. Contractions lasted 10–15 minutes.

A solution of rhubarb extract of the same strength was made. The optimal mixture in this case is 25 c.c. sea-water $+$ 0.5 c.c. or 1 c.c. rhubarb solution. In this mixture the contractions develop quickly and last 15 minutes or more.

[95] To appear shortly in Journal of Biological Chemistry.
[96] *Loc. cit.*

With aloin the concentration of the purgative needed to produce optimal results was somewhat greater than in cascara or rhubarb. Colocynth and podophyllin act similarly, but the contractions soon cease.

These vegetable purgatives thus act on the jellyfish, Polyorchis, in a way quite similar to that described by Loeb for saline purgatives.

Pilocarpine, though not used as a purgative on account of its special action on other organs of the body, has a powerful action also on the intestine. Its influence on the intestine is much like that of barium chloride. It causes violent contractions of the musculature of the gut and very active peristaltic movements. This is the case in whatever way the substance is administered. A few drops of a 1/10% solution of pilocarpine hydrochlorate in distilled water poured on the serous surfaces of the rabbit's intestine brings about almost immediately violent peristaltic movements. In addition to this there is an increase in the amount of fluid secreted into the intestine, 20–30 c.c. gathering in the small intestine in an hour. The evacuation of faeces takes place in about three-quarters of an hour. These may be of a semifluid character, and with larger doses resemble the faeces produced by $BaCl_2$. The antagonism between pilocarpine and $CaCl_2$ is incomplete. $CaCl_2$ is capable of inhibiting only temporarily the movements caused by pilocarpine.

It is interesting to note the marked purgative effect of pilocarpine in a small fresh-water crustacean (*Sida crystallina*). This animal, which has been spoken of in previous chapters belongs to the Cladocera. The intestine extends in a fairly straight line throughout the body, bending downward at the post abdomen to open to the outside. At the anterior end is a slight dilatation which may represent the stomach. From this there open two diverticula or coeca which seem to be of a glandular nature, and are sometimes spoken of as digestive glands. They are usually filled with a greenish fluid. The intestine is always filled with brown faeces which are normally expelled in small quantities, only at considerable intervals. Slight peristaltic waves are commonly seen in the lower part of the intestine.

These animals were placed in various solutions, and it was found[97] that pilocarpine hydrochlorate, aloin, cascara, as well as barium chloride, sodium citrate, sulphate, and fluoride, caused an increased peristaltic activity of the intestine, and a rapid expulsion of faeces, so that in a very short time the entire intestine was empty. At the same time the intestine becomes filled with a greenish fluid similar to that seen in the diverticula. This fluid may be also expelled and replaced again. It is evidently secreted by the intestine or by the diverticula as a result of the purgative action. Very dilute solutions of pilocarpine are sufficient to bring about this effect. In a 1% solution the action is very rapid, and evacuation of faeces may be brought about by a mixture of 1 c.c. 0.1% pilocarpine in 10 c.c. water. This takes place within 20 minutes.

An attempt was made to determine whether or not $CaCl_2$ is capable of inhibiting the action of pilocarpine. The experiments on rabbits in this respect were unsatisfactory. It was found that the greatest dilution at which expulsion of faeces in Sida could be caused in a short period of time was 1 c.c. 0.1% pilocarpine + 10 c.c. water. Animals were placed in a mixture of 1 c.c. 0.1% pilocarpine + 10 c.c. m/6 $CaCl_2$. These behaved exactly as though the water had not been replaced by $CaCl_2$. In other words, the presence of the $CaCl_2$ did not delay at all the action of the pilocarpine. This was repeated many times, and it seems that in Sida at least the action of pilocarpine is not at all antagonized by calcium chloride. In a mixture, however, of 10 c.c. 1% atropin sulphate + 1 c.c. 0.1% pilocarpine no evacnation of faeces took place and there was no increase in peristalsis.

[97] MacCallum, J. B.: University of California Publications, Vol. II, 1905, p. 65.

ND - #0013 - 300125 - C0 - 229/152/6 [8] - CB - 9780266262589 - Gloss Lamination